PREGNANCY
A GUIDE TO NATURAL THERAPIES

CHERYL BEALE

HILL OF CONTENT
Melbourne

First published in Australia 1999
by Hill of Content Publishing Co Pty Ltd
86 Bourke Street, Melbourne 3000
Tel: 03 9662 2282
Fax: 03 9662 2527
E-mail: hocpub@collinsbooks.com.au

© Copyright Cheryl Beale 1999

Cover design: Sonia Pletes and Graeme Moss

Editing and layout: Anna Tomlinson
Printed by: Australian Print Group, Maryborough Vic.

National Library of Australia
Cataloguing-in-Publication data

Beale, Cheryl, 1953 -
  Pregnancy: a guide to natural therapies

Includes index
ISBN 0 85572 294 0.

1. Pregnancy - Popular works. 2. Therapeutics,
Physiological. 3. Alternative medicine. I. Title.

618.24

This book gives information about the use of complementary therapies. This information is intended for education purposes only and is not intended to replace the advice of a qualified health professional. Consult your doctor about any medical condition.

CONTENTS

FOREWORD

Women today are seeking to take responsibility for their health and to work with their doctor to ensure the best possible outcome for their health. This is especially true during pregnancy when they wish to understand what is happening to their bodies. They wish to play an active role in their labour and birth. Obstetric practices have changed enormously over the past years in response to these demands. Birth Centres have evolved, women are encouraged to attend prenatal classes and support persons are active partners during labour and birth.

Our philosophy sees women taking active responsibility for their pregnancy. Birth Centres were developed for women who did not want an impersonal hospital experience for their birth. The mother works as part of a team with her doctor and her midwife. She is encouraged to care for herself during her pregnancy to support her own health and that of her baby. She is encouraged to learn about the process of labour and to take control of it.

Recognition of the role played by a variety of complementary therapies to support the mother's emotional and physical health is needed at a time of increased use of these therapies to maintain health while pregnant. There is considerable uncertainty about the appropriate use of many of these complementary therapies. To enable women to make informed decisions about their health care, Cheryl Beale has researched and presented information about a wide range of these therapies and their availability. The importance of a healthy diet, a healthy attitude, adequate exercise and plenty of fresh air cannot be overemphasised. Many minor but common complaints of pregnancy can be relieved using the simple measures recommended in this book. For example, aching backs can often be relieved with massage.

The best health care during pregnancy involves a team approach. This team will include an experienced and caring obstetrician and a capable and caring midwife, willing to spend time with the mother during her pregnancy and her labour. Knowledge and choice empower the mother, giving her the best opportunity to enjoy her pregnancy and to achieve a happy outcome. Complementary therapies can be used as a part of this approach to enrich a woman's experience through her pregnancy and into motherhood.

Dr Bruce Sutherland
Obstetrician
Hawthorn Birth Centre
Melbourne

SAFETY OF ESSENTIAL OILS, HERBS AND HOMOEOPATHIC PREPARATIONS DURING PREGNANCY AND LACTATION

Natural health care encompasses a wide range of therapeutic possibilities. The terms natural, holistic, complementary, alternative and traditional are often used interchangeably to refer to the field of health care that relies on a holistic view of the person rather than focusing on a disease state in isolation. The terms natural, holistic and traditional imply that these methods have been in use for many years, possibly for many centuries. This is certainly the case for acupuncture, herbalism and massage, all of which have many centuries of development and tradition behind their use. Homoeopathy, flower essences and essential oils have been in use for the past 150 years or less. Nutritional supplementation is a more recent therapeutic tool; many studies giving reliable nutritional information have been published in the past twenty years or so. Some good research was certainly available earlier, but the field is now growing at an enormous rate. There is currently a great deal of research being conducted by a number of organisations on the benefits of nutritional supplementation. The terms 'complementary' and, more recently, 'integrative' suggest that the two methods of medicine – orthodox and alternative – should work in cooperation for the best health outcomes for individual patients. There are many practitioners from both orthodox and alternative health fields working tirelessly to bring about understanding of, and cooperation between, each health paradigm. Many countries have government and private organisations responsible for developing protocols on the appropriate use of complementary forms of medicine.

Many universities and colleges are now offering postgraduate courses for orthodox medical practitioners to train in the various complementary fields. In many countries, nurses are actively involved in integrating complementary or holistic health care practices into mainstream medical care. Postgraduate courses are available through several colleges and universities. Some of these postgraduate courses are comprehensive, offering tuition in nutrition, the use of herbs, massage, relaxation and gentle exercise therapies such as yoga and tai chi. Holistic journals keep nurses up-to-date with information on new research into holistic and complementary therapies. America, Australia and England have well-established postgraduate holistic nursing courses and journals devoted to complementary health issues for nurses.

Herbal medicine has been used in almost every country of the world. Each country has relied on its unique plant life as a source of medicine. For example, China, India and Europe still use herbal medicine as an important aspect of their health care. Doctors in many European countries are trained in the use of herbs. The use of herbs is increasing in Australia, England and other countries as dissatisfaction grows with the side effects of strong pharmaceutical medicines and as the number of health complaints for which orthodox medicine can give no answer increases. The North American Indians have a powerful understanding of the medicinal properties of their native plants, many of which are now being used by people all over the world. Many of the herbs used in pregnancy and midwifery are native American herbs. In Australia, postgraduate courses in herbal medicine are now being offered for medical practitioners. Various associations and universities are funding studies into the efficacy and safety of herbs.

Acupuncture and homoeopathic medicine are widely practised in China and India respectively, and their popularity is spreading to many other countries. Both are being used as effective, simple, relatively inexpensive and safe alternatives to the use of synthetic drugs and invasive surgery. Doctors in England, Europe and Australia are studying these techniques and incorporating them into their practices. Similarly, nutritional medicine is also offered as a postgraduate course. Preventative or functional medicine, using nutritional measures to prevent disease, is gaining in popularity as many studies increasingly show the cost effectiveness of avoiding serious disease states. These measures include dietary manipulation as well as supplementation of specific nutrients. A large number of studies showing the benefits of nutritional supplementation and correct dietary choices in preventing ill-health, and in some cases reversing existing disease states, have been published by reputable medical journals.

The World Health Organisation (WHO) promotes the use of traditional forms of medicine and is engaged in integrating these into health care in many countries. The WHO recognises the importance and efficacy of many of these traditional practices and is developing guidelines for their use. The most important of these traditional practices are herbal medicine and acupuncture.

A major concern with these forms of medicine is whether they are safe to use, especially during pregnancy.

There is a great deal of misunderstanding about the safety of herbs, essential oils and vitamin supplements in pregnancy. All the recommendations in this book have been made using reputable sources as references. Many conditions can be easily prevented or controlled with some simple measures that have stood the test of time. Our modern health care system is based on crisis management rather than on the less expensive, less dramatic traditional health care systems of the past which were based on prevention using simple remedies with no side effects.

HERBS

There is a growing body of evidence for the safety and efficacy of herbs for many conditions. For reliable information on the use of herbs, it is appropriate to seek the recommendations of those who have a sound understanding of their modes of action. Australia, America and the World Health Organisation are currently developing monographs to document the chemistry, uses and contraindications for herbs used in those countries. The European Community has already published a number of monographs for some of the most widely available herbs. The European Scientific Cooperative on Phytotherapy (ESCOP), an international cooperative with 15 international scientific societies as members, established the ESCOP monographs. Commission E, an interdisciplinary expert body appointed by the Federal German Department of Health to register and prepare drugs for human use, has also established monographs on medicinal plants and herbs. Monographs on herbs are developed after extensive review of research conducted about the particular herb under investigation. Traditional uses are assessed and verified where possible. Safety data is analysed for each herb and all reported adverse effects are examined. If there is any possibility that the herb could be dangerous, this is noted in the monograph. Specific comment is made in each monograph about use during pregnancy and lactation. Many reported adverse effects have been found to be the result of mistaking one herb for another, often when the herb has been picked from the wild. This is a reminder to use herbs purchased only from reputable suppliers who guarantee strict quality control, and to use herbs strictly in the recommended dosages.

Many herbs have a long tradition of use during pregnancy and are known to be safe and effective. In this book I have recommended only herbs which have been researched well and found to be safe. The following herbs have been extensively reviewed and researched by different bodies established to monitor the safety and reliability of traditional herbs.

Herbs for Internal Use: chamomile flowers, dandelion root and herb, echinacea purpurea, garlic, ginger, hamamelis (witch-hazel), hops, horse chestnut, linseed, myrrh, passionflower herb, psyllium, St John's wort, and valerian.

Herbs for External Use: calendula flowers, chamomile flowers, and viola tricolor herb.

The other herbs mentioned in the book have a long tradition of use for the conditions described. This has been for some hundreds of years in the case of caulophyllum (blue cohosh), cimifuga (black cohosh), squaw vine, cramp bark, black haw, vitex agnus castus and echinacea angustifolia. Monographs for these have yet to be prepared, but they have a long history of safe use. According to the World Health Organisation (WHO), which advocates strongly the use of traditional healing modalities, the use of these herbs for the conditions indicated should rely on traditional recommendations. The use should be discontinued only where there is proof of adverse reaction. There have been no adverse reactions proven for the herbs recommended here in the many years of their use; thus, the recommendations in this book follow the WHO guidelines.

ESSENTIAL OILS

Many essential oils have a reputation for being dangerous during pregnancy. According to Robert Tisserand, an English aromatherapist who has done extensive research on essential oils and their safety and is regarded as an expert in the field of essential oil use, there is little evidence of possible dangers of many oils during pregnancy. On examination of the literature and research available, Tisserand found that many of the reported dangers resulted from the use of impure samples or from huge overdoses of the oils taken by mouth. In fact, he has also found that attempts to use essential oils to cause abortion have been unsuccessful. It is unfortunate that essential oils have gained such a poor reputation when it appears that it is largely undeserved.

However, Tisserand does suggest that some oils should be avoided as they may cross the placenta. These oils have not been used in this book. Nonetheless, I would like to stress how important it is to purchase only quality essential oils from a reputable supplier, and to use only one or two drops at any time. Never take essential oils internally – many of the reported dangers have come from ingestion of very large quantities in doses that could not be used normally. Do not substitute fragrant oils for essential oils.

The following list of safe oils has been compiled from the Commission E monographs and from research on toxicological reports by the Research Institute for Fragrance Materials, an English organisation which reports on safety testing of essential oils. The Institute also publishes data on toxicity, skin irritation and sensitivity and phototoxicity. These oils have been classified as safe and effective for external use during pregnancy, with no known associated toxicological problems: chamomile (Roman and German); clary sage; eucalyptus; geranium; lavender; neroli; patchouli; peppermint; petitgrain; pine needle; rose; and sandalwood.

A NOTE ABOUT CLARY SAGE

Clary sage is often recommended as appropriate only for use during labour. Its use during pregnancy is not recommended. However, according to Robert Tisserand, there is no reason to avoid its use during pregnancy. It is a very relaxing and anti-depressant oil and could be useful during pregnancy. It is also an easily available oil and not particularly expensive. However, as many authors continue to recommend against its use during pregnancy, I have chosen to follow this practice to avoid any confusion. Therefore, I have mentioned it only for use during labour and postnatally.

HOMOEOPATHY

In many countries homoeopathy is 150 years' old. It was also widely supported by the British royal family. Hospitals in the USA, the UK and Australia once dispensed homoeopathic remedies. Homoeopathy is still widely practised in many countries with many doctors now trained in its use.

Homoeopathic remedies are prepared using very small quantities of the active ingredient dispersed through a liquid such as water. This microscopic amount of the substance is then absorbed and utilised by the cells, correcting any imbalance in metabolism. These small amounts ensure that the remedies are safe as long as they are taken in the recommended dosages. If you self-prescribe homoeopathic remedies such as Arnica, take them only if you are experiencing the symptoms. Once your symptoms abate, stop taking the remedy.

TISSUE SALTS

Tissue salts are prepared homoeopathically and share the safety of homoeopathic remedies. Unlike homoeopathic remedies, however, there are only twelve tissue salts. These are available in health food stores. Like homoeopathic remedies, tissue salts are perfectly safe as long as you take them while you have some symptoms that match the remedy picture.

VITAMINS AND MINERALS

Numerous studies have shown the importance and efficacy of supplemental vitamins and minerals in pregnancy and for general health. Where possible, I have referred to the results of these studies. (For a complete list, however, please see the references section at the end of the book.)

Recommended values for individual nutrients are considerably less than the lowest levels associated with adverse reactions. These levels have been documented by the Australian Council for Responsible Nutrition, which has searched available literature to identify possible adverse reactions to doses of vitamins and minerals above the recommended daily intake (RDI). The Council has adopted a conservative value for its recommended lowest dosage.

The remedies discussed in this book should be taken only in the recommended doses and for the recommended conditions. If you have any doubt whatsoever about the use of a remedy, consult a trained naturopath, herbalist or homoeopath. Always seek appropriate medical help for severe problems or if the condition persists.

Finally, I have tried to write this book in a non-sexist way. Where it was not possible to use gender-neutral words, I have used the pronouns 'he' and 'his', particularly in reference to foetus and baby. This was done for purely practical reasons and is not meant to offend, exclude or denigrate. The comments in those cases apply equally to girls and boys.

HAPPY AND HEALTHY

Pregnancy should be a time of glowing good health, of joy and anticipation. Instead, the reality for many women is often much less harmonious. Plagued by fatigue, nausea, indigestion, sleepless nights, backache, constipation and mood swings, the pregnancy may be far less comfortable and joyful than expected. The physical and emotional demands of pregnancy can become overwhelming, especially if there are other children to be cared for, or if you are still pursuing a career.

A solid basis for a happy and healthy pregnancy involves three major aspects. You need each of the following in good supply: a healthy diet and nutrition, a healthy attitude and some sensible exercise.

A healthy diet supplies the rapidly growing foetus with the raw ingredients for its growth. If you feed your baby good, wholesome and nourishing food, he will have the ingredients to grow as healthy as possible. If you feed your baby take-away foods or food that is low in nutrition, the risk is that your child will miss out on some important ingredients necessary for his best growth and development. As nature intends the unborn child to have the best nutrition possible for his growth, you may suffer nutritional deficiencies as the child will be nourished from your reserves. This can lead to your body losing essential nutrients. For example, calcium may be withdrawn from your bones, leading to potential dental problems or osteoporosis later in life. If there are insufficient nutrients in your reserves, the baby will miss out. This might lead to only minor problems which may never be detected, or it could be much more severe. For example, lack of folic acid can lead to spina bifida, high pesticide exposure before and during pregnancy has been implicated in attention deficit disorder and hyperactivity, and low levels of vitamin A may contribute to cleft palate.

The mental and emotional aspects of pregnancy are often overlooked. The emphasis is generally placed on the physical changes, which are obvious and are more easily explained and managed. While physical health in pregnancy is extremely important, so too are emotional wellbeing and mental attitude. There are huge emotional changes during pregnancy as a result of hormonal fluctuations. There are also lifestyle changes as a result of the demands of pregnancy and the subsequent arrival of a new family member. Many of us overwork and rarely find time to nurture ourselves. Many women disregard the demands of pregnancy and expect that it will make no difference to their energy levels, career pursuits or other obligations. Many women are disappointed with themselves if they cannot keep up with their usual schedules and routines, or if they find themselves more emotional than usual.

Our thoughts as well as our physical health affect the unborn child. Our fears and our frights will be transmitted. Just as the umbilical cord, the baby's lifeline, provides food and nourishment, so it is also a source of love and nurturing for the child. With a good, healthy attitude you will find necessary time for yourself. Recognise the changing circumstances of your life. Make sure that you get plenty of rest and relaxation, and adequate sleep. You might listen to satisfying music, treat yourself to a regular massage and regularly practise some yoga or meditation. Send your child loving, comforting messages. Play comforting and pleasant music, talk to your child and encourage your partner and other children to do the same. Babies respond to sounds and voices which they have heard during their time in the womb. Familiar music is calming and familiar voices are soothing to babies, to children and to adults.

Exercise is known to improve your feeling of wellbeing, to improve sleep, and to keep muscles toned and strengthened. Healthy exercise during pregnancy should be moderate and comfortable. Do not start a vigorous exercise program during pregnancy. Never raise your heart rate, your breathing rate or your body temperature above comfortable levels. Stretching exercises, walking, swimming, tai chi, or gentle water aerobics specially designed for pregnancy could be considered. Get plenty of fresh air. If you are not sure whether an exercise program is appropriate or if you have any particular health problems, check with your doctor or with a physiotherapist who specialises in exercise for pregnancy. Appropriate exercise has been used in gestational diabetes and in Type II diabetes to maintain blood sugar levels. If you have any tendency to diabetes, discuss this with your doctor, as a specially developed exercise program may improve your general health during your pregnancy.

With healthy nutrition, healthy attitude and appropriate exercise as a basis for your good health in pregnancy, you will avoid many of the usual complaints and problems. Generally you will sleep better, you will have adequate energy while recognising your increased need for rest, and you will understand your mood changes and nurture yourself through them. You should experience less constipation and fewer aches and pains.

Unfortunately, in spite of your best efforts, there may still be some discomforts or problems. Many of these complaints of pregnancy are often regarded as relatively minor, although they may not seem so at the time. These minor problems do not have to be an integral part of pregnancy and you do not have to put up with them. Many can be dealt with easily and safely. Naturopathy, nutritional therapies, acupuncture, homoeopathy, massage and osteopathy all offer a number of safe and proven suggestions to help you overcome many of the discomforts of pregnancy.

Pregnancy is also a time of preparation for the experience of labour and childbirth. Keeping yourself well and healthy during pregnancy is an important part of your overall plan for a speedy, efficient and manageable labour. You will approach labour and birth prepared and in good health. This will give your child the best possible start in life. You will start motherhood in the best possible health, with improved energy levels and well-established patterns of caring for and nurturing yourself, your partner and your child.

Chapter 1

GROWTH AND DEVELOPMENT

The changes occurring during foetal growth are the most profound of any stage of human development. During pregnancy, the embryo develops from a single fertilised egg to a fully formed and functioning individual with unique characteristics. A pregnancy will last, on average, nine lunar months or about 266 days. While huge technological advances have made it possible for parents to see an ultrasound picture of their baby, there is much that remains unknown about any particular child. Only when the child has been born can the parents have a realistic view of him or her. Only as the child grows and matures can personality and individual traits be identified.

During the mother's pregnancy, hormonal changes result in many physical changes necessary for the survival of the baby before and after birth. Many of these changes are obvious, such as the growth of the abdomen with the increasing size of the baby. Others are less obvious, but nevertheless important, such as relaxation of ligaments, food cravings and sore breasts.

Table 1 gives a guide to the development of the pregnancy and of the baby. The timing is based on a 40-week pregnancy, with the first day of your last period being counted as the start of week 1. This means that you are not pregnant until sometime during week 3. Different pregnancies may develop at different rates, especially during the second half of the pregnancy, so the times given here are considered to be average times. If you have an ultrasound, you will be given an estimate of the duration of the pregnancy and an expected due date for delivery. These ultrasound dates are considered to be accurate to within seven to ten days, which means that the due date is a guide only. Many midwives consider the normal length of a pregnancy to be between thirty-seven and forty-two weeks.

Table 1.   Development and Changes in Mother and Baby During Pregnancy

WEEK	MOTHER	BABY
1	last period	
2		
3	ovulation	conception
4		implantation
	breasts may feel tender	now called an embryo
	missed period	placenta develops
		brain forms two lobes
		about 2 mm long
	may need to urinate frequently	
6	nausea and morning sickness	limb buds appear
	may have dizziness and faintness	spinal cord and brain
	nodules appear on areolae	tiny fingers and toes
	nipples may be more prominent	circulation starts
		heart begins to beat
8	nausea continues	
	cravings	palate and upper lip develop
	easily fatigued	ears and eyes form
		baby moves about
		about 1.3 cm long
10	uterus is the size of an orange	fingers and toes obvious
		the heart functions
12	uterus now above the level of the pubis	now called a foetus
	morning sickness usually passes	face appears more human
		about 6.5 cm long
14	less easily fatigued	eyebrows and some hair develop
	dark line may form down the centre of the abdomen	passes urine into the amniotic fluid
	nipples may darken	
16	may perspire more readily	fully formed
		maturity and growth continue
		lanugo (fine hair) forms
		sex identifiable
		about 16 cm long
18	increasing weight around waist and hips	heart beat audible
	may start to be aware of movement	may suck thumb
		about 20 cm long

20	uterus may press against lungs and stomach may have heartburn, indigestion and reflux navel may protrude	vernix forms to protect skin moves about freely
22	Braxton Hicks contractions may start gums may swell with hormonal effects	fingernails form becomes very active during the mother's sleep
	uterus reaches the umbilicus	
24	the top of the uterus reaches above the navel may experience cramps	eyes partly open heart can be easily heard through a stethoscope
	pressure on bladder starts to increase	veins may be visible through the skin about 32 cm long, 0.5 kg vernix covers entire body
26	stretch marks may become visible	can hear your voice eyes open
28	colostrum may leak	heart reacts to mother's voice about 38 cm long, 0.9 kg able to hiccup
30	less room in uterus, movement more obvious may become breathless on exertion	fat layers forming usually head down testes descend about 42 cm long, 1.8 kg
34	ligaments and muscles continue to relax in preparation for birth may experience backache	able to differentiate light and dark about 44 cm long, 2.5 kg
38	if pregnancy is a first, baby may lighten with greater comfort and easier breathing amniotic fluid renewed every 3 hours cervix softens	may practise breathing swallows amniotic fluid increasing weight bowels filled with green or black meconium from the digestive organs has firm grasp lanugo almost gone kidneys and lungs mature
40	due date	fingernails overlap fingertips testes in scrotum or in inguinal canals

Chapter 2

NUTRITION DURING PREGNANCY

We are dependent on various nutrients for a healthy life. We need to obtain these regularly in our diets or we set ourselves up for sickness. Many of today's common illnesses are diet related. For example, heart disease, obesity and some cancers are known to be directly related to our modern diet.

Pregnancy especially is a time of heightened nutritional requirements. The growing child has his own unique nutritional needs and the mother needs extra nutrition for the growing uterus and placenta. A good diet and healthy nutrition form an important part of the basis for a healthy pregnancy. As adequate nutrition before and during pregnancy is so vital, a complete chapter is devoted to helping you understand the role of various essential nutrients. There is, unfortunately, a good deal of misunderstanding about what constitutes a healthy diet. Many people are confused about the safety of, and the need for, extra supplements and about the requirements of some important nutrients such as calcium.

The first part of this chapter deals in some detail with nutrition and the basis of a healthy diet. If you find this section heavy going, skip to the recommended diet towards the end of the chapter. Recommendations for appropriate supplements are included at the very end of this chapter.

The essential nutrients for good health will be discussed under a few headings to give you a better understanding of how and why a healthy diet is vital to your own health and the health of your child. This will also help you to plan your diet during your pregnancy and postnatal period. The important nutrients to be discussed are: carbohydrates, proteins, fats and oils, vitamins and minerals.

To help you understand the amounts of each type of food needed in your diet, have a look at the food pyramid. Fruits and vegetables, and breads and cereals make up the base of the pyramid. Similarly, they should make up the basis of your daily diet. These foods constitute the group known as carbohydrates.

The Food Pyramid Chart

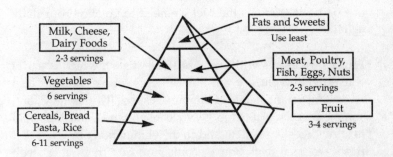

Size of Servings in Food Pyramid

Food	Size of One Serving
Bread	1 slice
Pasta	$^1/_2$ cup of cooked pasta
Rice	$^1/_2$ cup of cooked rice
Cereal	1 cup of cold ready-to-eat cereal **or** $^1/_2$ cup of cooked cereal
Vegetables	$^1/_2$ cup of cooked or raw vegetables **or** 1 cup of leafy vegetables
Fruit	1 piece of fruit or equivalent wedge of watermelon etc. $^1/_2$ cup canned/stewed fruit $^1/_4$ cup dried fruit
Low fat milk	1 cup
Low fat yoghurt	1 cup
Low fat cottage cheese	45g ($1^1/_2$ oz) natural or 60g (2 oz) processed
Fish	100g (3 oz)
Lean meat or skinless chicken	100g (3 oz)
Egg	1 egg

CARBOHYDRATES

Carbohydrates fall into four main groups: fruits, vegetables, grains or cereals, and legumes. Their major job is to provide energy in the form of glucose. This is the main sugar used by our bodies to give us the fuel we need to go about our daily activities.

Fruits provide us with fructose (fruit sugar), which is easily converted into glucose, our major energy source. They are also a very important source of vitamins, especially vitamin C, and some minerals. Fruits are very cleansing and contribute to a healthy digestive system and to the elimination of wastes. Eat fresh, seasonal fruit. Some people find that they digest fruit more easily if they eat it alone with no other food in the stomach about twenty minutes or so before a meal. This can be especially true of melons.

Vegetables supply us with vitamins, minerals, some protein, starch and chlorophyll. Starches are converted into glucose by a number of enzymes in our digestive system. This process begins with saliva in the mouth. Therefore, it is important that we chew our food thoroughly. This breaks the food into small pieces to enable the enzymes in saliva to start the process of digestion more easily.

Many of us regard vegetables as secondary and often unpleasant adjuncts on our dinner plates. You will find them more enjoyable if you experiment with different vegetables. Buy yourself a cookbook which shows you simple ways to cook and enjoy them. Try making fresh vegetable juices. This maximises the availability of nutrients as they are easily digested in this form. Don't mix vegetable and fruit juices. They are best taken separately.

Grains, or cereals, supply us with energy, protein, vitamins and minerals, and are low in fat. Only the whole grain which has not been processed or refined contains all the goodies. Brown rice and wholegrain bread are much better for you than their refined counterparts. Experiment with barley, corn, millet and oats to give yourself plenty of variety and a wide range of nutrients.

Legumes, or pulses, are probably the least understood of the carbohydrate foods. As well as providing us with carbohydrates, they are an important source of protein. They include chickpeas, soy beans, lentils, lima beans, kidney beans, aduki beans, broad beans, green beans and peas. Peanuts are also legumes, they are not true nuts.

Legumes also supply minerals and vitamins in an easily absorbable form. Sprouts from the mung bean, known as bean sprouts or bean shoots, and other sprouts are high in very easily absorbable protein, minerals and vitamins.

Use a cookbook and experiment with a different legume each week. Lentils and other beans are used in Indian cookery. Chickpeas and sesame paste (tahini) form the basis of hommos (sometimes spelt hummus), a Lebanese dip. Tofu is prepared from soy beans and is used in Chinese cookery. Minestrone and many vegetable soup recipes contain beans.

Fibre is classed as a carbohydrate, but one which is not digested. It does not provide us with vitamins, calories or other nutrients, but has other important roles. The benefits of fibre occur mostly in the digestive tract. Fibre is of two types – soluble and insoluble. Soluble fibre helps remove fats and cholesterol from your system, and absorbs water in your digestive tract. This has the effect of slowing digestion in your stomach so that you feel satisfied for longer. It helps maintain stable blood sugar levels, which means that you will not constantly crave sweet foods such as chocolate. Soluble fibre is found in legumes, cabbage and many fruits. Insoluble fibre has the job of speeding food through your system so that it doesn't sit around for too long. It acts as a broom to sweep food through your system. This reduces the time that toxic products stay in your digestive system and their consequent absorption across the intestinal wall. Insoluble fibre is found in bran, in other cereals and in many vegetables.

Many studies have shown that increased dietary fibre decreases the risk of a wide range of common health problems. These include constipation, diabetes, obesity, colon cancer, heart disease, and high blood pressure. To increase your fibre intake you need to increase both types of fibre. The best way to do this is to eat a variety of fibre-containing foods. A diet high in fruit, vegetables and whole grains will give you a balance of both types of fibre. Bran is a reasonable source of insoluble fibre, but also use some soluble fibres such as oat bran, linseed and psyllium. If you are easily constipated, you need to increase both types of fibre, not just bran.

PROTEINS

Protein is essential for growth and tissue repair. Protein is actually a combination of amino acids. There are several amino acids. Some of these are essential, which means that our bodies need to obtain them from our diets every day. Adults need eight essential amino acids, while babies and children need ten. (The essential amino acids are: isoleucine, leucine, lysine, methionine, phenylalanine, threonine, tryptophan and valine. Babies and children also need histidine and arginine in their diets.) Provided the body has adequate quantities of the essential amino acids, it can synthesise some other amino acids, called non-essential amino acids.

Protein is digested by enzymes in various parts of the digestive system, but relies on being chewed into small particles so that the maximum surface area is presented for enzyme activity. These particles are broken down by the enzymes into smaller and smaller chains of amino acids called peptides, and then into individual amino acids to be absorbed by the blood stream.

Generally two or three small serves of protein should be eaten each day. As you digest only a small amount of protein at any meal, it is preferable to have several small serves rather than one large serve at one meal. Protein foods include dairy foods, poultry and eggs, meat and fish, grains, legumes, nuts and seeds. Eggs and fish provide the most easily digestible forms of protein.

Nuts and Seeds

Nuts provide all the essential amino acids, minerals (notably calcium and magnesium), vitamin B and vitamin E. A combination of almonds, brazil nuts and cashews provides a complete protein. Nuts may be high in fats, but they are of the unsaturated variety (see the section on fats for more information on saturated and unsaturated fats). They also provide essential fatty acids.

Seeds are a neglected food in our society. Choose from pumpkin, sesame and sunflower. Seeds provide a complete protein as well as vitamins A and B, and minerals such as iron (especially in pumpkin seeds) and calcium (especially in sesame seeds). Sesame seeds are made into tahini, an easily digestible paste which can be used as a spread and is an ingredient in hommos.

Alfalfa and mung bean sprouts are seeds which have been sprouted to provide an easily digestible food, full of protein, vitamins and minerals. Many types of sprouts are commonly available wherever you buy your fruits and vegetables. They all provide a good and easily digestible source of nutrients.

Legumes

Legumes are both a protein food and a carbohydrate food and have been described in the section on carbohydrates. Beans, lentils and peas are legumes. As sources of protein they contain some or all of the essential amino acids in easily digestible forms. Used as a substitute for animal protein a couple of times a week, they can reduce the incidence of heart disease associated with the overconsumption of animal proteins. Soy beans are the only legume which contains all the essential amino acids and forms a complete protein. Other legumes need to be combined to give a complete range of the essential amino acids required for a complete protein. If you are having legumes, combine them with each other, or with grains. For example, have lentils and rice or baked beans on toast. Combinations of legume with legume or legume with grain will give you a complete protein.

Dairy Foods

Milk contains large amounts of calcium and protein. Unfortunately, for many of us cow's milk is extremely difficult to digest. The enzymes required to digest milk gradually deteriorate during early childhood. Also, for many people, milk is a highly allergic food causing mucus build up, stomach cramps, bloating, and rashes, to name a few reactions. Goat's milk, soy milk and milks prepared from oats, rice and sesame seeds generally cause fewer reactions.

Yoghurt is a milk product containing enzymes which help in its digestion. Many people find that they can tolerate yoghurt, but not other forms of milk products. Choose natural yoghurt with no added fruit. These yoghurts contain lactobacillus acidophilus and bifidus, which are beneficial bacteria in your digestive system. Fruit yoghurts have been sweetened and often do not contain adequate amounts of these bacteria. Add fresh fruit yourself if you like fruit yoghurt.

Cheese is also digestible by some people who cannot tolerate milk. Cheese provides calcium and protein, and hard cheeses provide vitamin A. Avoid processed cheeses. Some people find that they can tolerate the hard cheeses, but have difficulties with the moulds on softer cheeses.

Eggs have been unfairly maligned in the past. They are a very good source of easily digestible protein, and contain some vitamin A and B as well as iron. They were avoided due to their high cholesterol content. But eggs also contain lecithin, a substance which converts fats and cholesterol into tiny particles which can be metabolised by your body. Boiled or poached eggs are better than eggs cooked with butter or fat. Obtain free-range eggs from a health food store, as they are better for you nutritionally and taste much better than battery-produced eggs.

Poultry

Chicken is the most popular of the poultry foods available, but turkey, duck and geese add variety to your diet. Similarly to eggs, free-range produce is better for you and tastes much better. Free-range poultry generally contains fewer build-ups of antibiotics and artificial hormones. The use of antibiotics in our poultry and meat supplies has been implicated in the development of bacteria resistant to antibiotics.

Chicken has less available protein than nuts, legumes and fish, but is still a reasonable source. All poultry provides a complete protein except turkey. Turkey does not contain tryptophan and is therefore not a complete protein, but as it is eaten only occasionally this is not generally of concern.

Seafood

Fish provides a very easily digestible protein, but is not eaten often enough in Australia. Fatty fishes such as tuna, salmon, sardines, trout and mackerel contain essential fatty acids called omega-3 fatty acids. These have been found to lower cholesterol; protect against heart disease; benefit migraine, arthritis and psoriasis sufferers; and balance hormone levels; and are vital for brain and nervous system development.

Good quality fresh fish is becoming more easily available. Don't use processed, packaged or frozen fish. Don't fry it or use batter because your meal then becomes full of saturated fat and contains much less of the goodness you need.

Unfortunately, many people dislike or are allergic to shell-fish. Shellfish is a valuable source of chromium and other minerals for those who enjoy it and are not allergic to it. Shellfish used to be regarded as a food high in cholesterol, but it now appears that the levels of cholesterol it contains are equivalent to those found in chicken, beef and other meats.

Meat

Meat is generally more difficult to digest than other forms of protein foods. For this reason, it is not as good a source of protein as fish or eggs, but it is still able to supply us with adequate amounts of protein and some other nutrients, notably iron, magnesium and the B vitamins. It is not useful as a source of most other minerals or the vitamins A and C. Eaten in moderation, meat supplies a variety of both taste and nutrition.

The problem with meat arises when large amounts of it are eaten and it is the main focus of a meal. Saturated fats and cholesterol usually accompany meat. These are discussed more fully in the section on fats, but eating less animal fat has been shown in numerous studies to lower the risk of heart disease and other nasties. Meat also absorbs many of the pesticides used in the animal's food, and many of the chemical additives and artificial hormones used in the growth of the animal and in the preparation of the meat for the consumer.

Whenever you eat meat, remove the visible fat, have small amounts only and ensure that you also have lots of fresh vegetables with the meal. This will help your body get the best out of your food and ensure that you obtain a good balance of nutrients.

FATS AND OILS

Fats and oils, referred to as lipids, are at the top of the food pyramid. This means that your diet should contain only small amounts of them. The problem is generally in trying to keep your intake to a minimum, rather than trying to get enough. Fats and oils supply us with energy, the fat-soluble vitamins A, D and E, and essential fatty acids. In cold climates, fat deposits protect us from the cold. Fats in a meal also take longer to digest than the rest of the meal, leaving us feeling full and satisfied for longer.

Fats are usually solids at room temperature and are found in animal products such as meat and butter. Oils are usually liquid at room temperature.

Cholesterol is one of the best known of the fats. All animals produce cholesterol and all animal produce contains cholesterol. It is a complex type of lipid made by the liver and stored in the liver. We make sufficient cholesterol for our needs.

Cholesterol is vital for cell membranes and the nervous system, and is an essential part of a number of hormones, including oestrogen. It combines with a number of other substances to form bile, which is stored by the gall bladder until it is needed to help with the digestion of fats and oils. While we need some cholesterol in our bodies, too much can lead to deposits in our blood vessels and the condition known as atherosclerosis or hardening of the arteries. Cholesterol combines with low density lipoproteins (LDLs), which are taken up by the body's cells as an energy source. After use by the cells, the cholesterol must then be returned to the liver by the high density lipoproteins (HDLs). Therefore, high levels of HDLs will reduce the risk of heart and artery disease and obesity by removing the cholesterol from the area. HDLs also transport the fat-soluble vitamins A, D and E. A high cholesterol level is good if the cholesterol is of the HDL variety, but it is dangerous if it is of the LDL variety. Exercise and a diet high in omega-6 and especially omega-3 fatty acids will help lower overall cholesterol levels. Omega-3 fatty acids are contained in fish oils, cod liver oil and linseed oil. Omega-6 fatty acids are found in sunflower, safflower and evening primrose oils. The vitamins C and E, and adequate amounts of lecithin in our bodies, can protect the blood vessel walls from accumulating cholesterol deposits. Smoking and diets high in animal fats, coconut oil and sugar contribute to high levels of LDLs. Contrary to popular opinion, most shellfish are not high in cholesterol and have been found to contain amounts equivalent to those in chicken and beef.

Animal products such as butter, milk, beef and lamb also contain saturated fats. These saturated fats are not essential for health and contribute to high cholesterol levels.

Polyunsaturated fats are found in vegetable sources and are the main source of the three essential fatty acids – linoleic, linolenic and arachidonic acids. Omega-3 fatty acids contained in fish oils and linseed oil are polyunsaturated fats. These oils have been mentioned earlier in their role of protecting against heart disease. They are also important in reducing inflammation due to skin problems such as dry skin, eczema and psoriasis, and in arthritic conditions. Any of these conditions suggest a need for increased omega-3 fatty acids.

When using polyunsaturated oils, use only cold pressed oils. Cold pressed oils contain vitamin E. This important vitamin is destroyed when oils are heated. While polyunsaturated fats are good for us, once they are heated they are converted to trans-fatty acids, which are not good for us. In fact, trans-fatty acids are carcinogenic, that is, they have been implicated in causing cancer. They can also act as saturated fats and stimulate the production of cholesterol. Margarine often contains high levels of these trans-fatty acids.

Monounsaturated fats actually decrease cholesterol levels. These fats are found in olive oil and nuts. Most natural foods provide a range of monounsaturated and polyunsaturated fats. Cold pressed oils such as olive, safflower, sunflower, avocado, soy, wheat germ and sesame provide us with a wide variety of polyunsaturated and monounsaturated fats. They also provide vitamin E. Sunflower oil provides vitamin D, which is necessary for calcium absorption. Coconut oil, which is used in many processed foods, is high in saturated fat, and its use should be minimised.

VITAMINS

Vitamin A

Vitamin A is a fat-soluble vitamin. It is necessary for good eyesight, for healthy skin and for the tissues lining your respiratory tract. Often lacking in asthmatics, supplemental vitamin A can protect the delicate lining of the airways against pollutants. It is one of the antioxidant vitamins which deactivate free radicals. These are unstable compounds formed in the body which may injure normal cells. They are a product of polluting chemicals in our atmosphere, such as pesticides, cigarette smoke and petrol fumes. Vitamin A deficiency has been linked to kidney and gall stones.

Vitamin A is available in two forms. Preformed vitamin A, or retinol, is contained in fish and especially fish oils. Cod liver and halibut oils are excellent sources of preformed vitamin A. Provitamin A is found in red, yellow and green vegetables, and is converted to vitamin A by the body. Beta carotene is available as a provitamin A supplement, but it should not be taken in isolation. If you take beta carotene as a supplement, make sure you also take the other antioxidants, vitamins C and E.

There has been a great deal of misinformation about vitamin A. Very high doses have been linked to foetal abnormalities. The potentially damaging doses were as high as 25,000 iu to 500,000 iu. These levels are much higher than you would normally be exposed to, even if you take a vitamin A supplement. Levels of 6000 iu have been used in a number of studies to reduce the risk of defects such as cleft palate and to prevent habitual miscarriage. Smokers with low levels of vitamin C and vitamin A in amniotic fluid are more likely to have preterm rupture of foetal membranes.

The B Vitamins

These work as a team and are better taken together rather than as individuals, except for short periods of time. Many people obtain less than the daily requirement for the B vitamins. Vitamin B1 has often been found to be deficient during pregnancy. Relative deficiencies of B vitamins can occur if you take large doses of a single B vitamin for any length of time. Many of the B vitamins are found in whole grains, but our practice of using processed flour and white rice has removed many of the B vitamins from our food supply. The birth control pill depletes B vitamins. If you conceive without making up these losses, you need to increase your intake during your pregnancy.

The B vitamins include vitamin B1 (thiamine), vitamin B2 (riboflavin), vitamin B3 (niacin or niacinamide), vitamin B5 (pantothenic acid), vitamin B6 (pyridoxine), vitamin B12 (cobalamin) and folic acid. Most of them are not stored by the body and need to be included in the diet every day.

The B vitamins help with metabolising our sources of carbohydrates, proteins and fats and converting them to energy. They are necessary to help us deal with stress and lack of the B vitamins has been implicated in some forms of depression. They help us produce antibodies against disease. They are essential for healthy skin, hair and eyes, and for a good memory. Vitamin B3 is necessary for the production of male and female hormones.

B vitamins are found in meat, fish, whole grains, nuts and seeds.

Vitamin B12 is a little different to the other members of the B family. It is mostly obtained from meat, fish and eggs, which means that strict vegetarians need to take a supplement. It is also found in brewer's yeast and mushrooms. Only small amounts are needed and B12 is stored in the body for long periods of time, so a deficiency may not be obvious for a number of years. A deficiency of vitamin B12 is known as pernicious anaemia.

Folic acid has derived its name from the word foliage, as it is contained in abundant amounts in green leafy vegetables. It is also found in liver and legumes. It is needed for healthy red blood cells and for the absorption of iron and calcium. Deficiencies of folic acid have been linked with neural tube defects in babies, a type of anaemia and infertility. Supplementation with folic acid is recommended during the months before you conceive and for the first three months of pregnancy to avoid neural tube defects.

Biotin, Inositol and Choline

Much less is known about these three B vitamins. They are important for the nervous system, in the breakdown of fats and protein, in the reduction of cholesterol, and in keeping skin and hair healthy. They can be found in liver, eggs, whole grains and brewer's yeast.

Vitamin C

We need to obtain our vitamin C every day. It is quickly processed through our bodies and is rapidly destroyed by heat. It is essential for healthy skin, ligaments and bones. It is another antioxidant vitamin protecting us against environmental pollutants, and has been used to protect against frequent colds. Large amounts of vitamin C are used whenever we are under stress and so extra vitamin C is beneficial whenever we are ill, busy or not getting sufficient sleep. This is one of the reasons it is vital to eat plenty of fresh fruits and vegetables when we are sick, overworked or stressed in any way. Smokers with low levels of vitamin C and vitamin A in amniotic fluid are more likely to have preterm rupture of foetal membranes. The birth control pill depletes B vitamins and vitamin C. If you conceive without making up these losses, you need to increase your intake during pregnancy.

Fresh fruit, especially citrus fruits, and raw vegetables supply us with most of our vitamin C. Vitamin C is also known as ascorbic acid, but in supplements it can be found as calcium ascorbate or sodium ascorbate. The best forms of supplemental vitamin C include bioflavonoids, which potentiate its action.

Vitamin D

Vitamin D is produced by the action of sunlight on the skin and is a fat-soluble vitamin, like vitamins A and E. It is best known for its regulation of mineral metabolism, especially calcium. Rickets disease, which affects the bones of some children who live in cold climates, is caused by a lack of vitamin D. Vitamin D is available in cod liver oil, egg yolks, salmon, herring and sardines.

Vitamin E

Also known as alpha tocopherol, vitamin E is the third of the antioxidant trio. With vitamins A and C, vitamin E has been shown to reduce the risk of a variety of cancers and to improve cardiovascular health. It increases levels of the good fats in your body, the HDLs. It helps maintain the normal blood supply via the umbilical cord to the unborn child. Vitamin E is found in cold pressed oils, wheat germ, eggs and leafy green vegetables. If you need to take a supplement, always start with low doses of vitamin E, 100 iu, and build up to higher doses as your body gets used to it.

Vitamin K

Vitamin K is required for the conversion of carbohydrates into usable sources of energy. It is important for blood clotting, for the functioning of the circulatory system and protects against the lead in exhaust fumes. Vitamin K can be found in soy beans, in dark green and leafy vegetables, especially lettuce, and in alfalfa.

ESSENTIAL FATTY ACIDS

Essential fatty acids include omega-3 and omega-6 fatty acids. The omega-3 essential fatty acids we need are alpha-linolenic acid (sometimes referred to as linolenic acid), EPA (eicosapentaenoic acid) and DHA (docosahhexaenoic acid). Fish oils contain omega-3 fatty acids, which have been found to lower cholesterol and triglyceride levels. You may have seen supplements containing EPA and DHA. These are made from fish oils and provide some of the omega-3 fatty acids.

The omega-6 fatty acids are linoleic, gamma-linolenic and arachidonic acids. Collectively, the omega-6 fatty acids are known as vitamin F.

Deficiencies of any of the essential fatty acids may contribute to dry skin and eczema. Supplementation with fatty acids in the form of fish oils and evening primrose oil has been found to reduce migraine in some sufferers, to relieve arthritis and to reduce the scaling of psoriasis. Fish oils have been used to lower blood pressure.

Eat plenty of wheat germ, nuts and seeds, legumes and fish, and use cold pressed oils such as safflower and sunflower, to maintain healthy levels of essential fatty acids.

MINERALS

Minerals are a vital part of our diet. They are often forgotten in the nutrient debate as the focus tends to be on vitamins. Due to our farming practices, our food does not contain the levels of minerals that it should or that we think it does. As many of us are living longer and becoming subject to the ravages of osteoporosis and other diet-related diseases, it is vital that we obtain adequate amounts of minerals before we start to exhibit overt disease.

Calcium is the major mineral in our body. It is required for healthy bones and teeth, for the muscles of the digestive tract and for the heart. Most of our calcium is in our bones. Calcium is a very difficult mineral to digest and needs magnesium, phosphorus and vitamins A, C and D to function effectively. Deficiencies of calcium during pregnancy have been linked with toxaemia of pregnancy and with high blood pressure. Calcium is needed to help prevent viral infections and helps reduce fatigue.

Requirements for calcium increase enormously during pregnancy and lactation. The baby will take calcium at the expense of the mother if there is a shortage. It will be withdrawn from the bones, the hair and the teeth; hence the expression, "For every baby, a tooth". This loss of teeth does not need to occur if there is adequate calcium in the diet and in a supplement, if necessary.

Calcium-rich foods include dairy foods, sardines and salmon (especially the bones), green leafy vegetables, oysters, nuts and seeds. Eat plenty of sesame seeds, almonds and brazil nuts. Chocolate and coffee can interfere with calcium metabolism as can table salt, alcohol and diets high in fats.

Chromium is vital for the utilisation of sugars and helps the body to maintain normal blood glucose levels. It is therefore useful for diabetics. It can be found in shellfish, meat, chicken, whole grains and some vegetables.

The chromium content of white blood cells decreases by as much as fifty per cent during pregnancy. This may explain partly the incidence of gestational diabetes and intolerance to alcohol during pregnancy. Low chromium levels may be found whenever the diet is high in processed carbohydrates.

Iron is necessary for a healthy blood supply and the increase in blood volume during pregnancy calls for extra iron. This is usually recommended by most doctors. But also avoid coffee and tea as these affect iron absorption. Your iron supplement should also contain vitamin C as this helps iron absorption. If your supplement causes constipation or diarrhoea, take a tissue salt called Ferrum Phos with it. (See chapter 10 for further details on the tissue salts and how to use them.) This helps your body absorb and metabolise the iron. Anaemia caused by iron deficiency is associated with a higher rate of premature birth.

Good natural sources of iron include green vegetables, kelp, sesame and pumpkin seeds, and meat.

Magnesium is an often neglected mineral, which works with calcium for strong bones and teeth. It is needed for the heart and a deficiency can contribute to high blood pressure. It has been suggested that many people get less than three-quarters of the recommended daily allowance (RDA) of magnesium. This is particularly worrying when you learn that magnesium deficiency has been implicated in the genesis of osteoporosis. The emphasis on the role of calcium has been at the expense of magnesium. Excess consumption of dairy foods can produce a magnesium deficiency. The current fad of recommending calcium without magnesium may be doing many women a great disservice.

Sources of magnesium include green leafy vegetables, wheat bran, whole grains, bananas, sesame seeds, cashews, brazil nuts and walnuts.

Magnesium is very difficult to absorb from our diet, and is rapidly being depleted in our soil. The need for magnesium increases by at least fifty per cent in the last trimester of pregnancy. Diets high in fat prevent magnesium absorption. Magnesium supplementation has been shown to decrease the severity of leg cramps in pregnancy. Low birth weight babies have greater survival rates and less risk of cerebral palsy if the mother is supplemented with magnesium during the pregnancy.

Manganese is another often forgotten mineral. It is vital for bone structure, for digestion, and for the production of milk in lactating women. It has been useful for diabetics and for combating fatigue. Manganese is found in shellfish, nuts, green leafy vegetables and whole grains.

Molybdenum, another neglected mineral, helps with carbohydrate and fat metabolism and works with iron in preventing anaemia. Tooth enamel contains a large amount of molybdenum and cavities may be due to low levels in the diet. It is found in whole grains, legumes and sunflower seeds.

Phosphorus is needed to help transport fatty acids about, for the metabolism of protein and carbohydrates, for the nervous system, and for the heart and circulation. In its best-known role it works with calcium to develop our bones. Excess sugar can prevent absorption of phosphorus, as can the use of antacids. Phosphorus is found in nuts and seeds, whole grains, fish, meat, poultry, eggs, cheese and many common food additives.

Potassium works with sodium to regulate the water balance in your body. It also regulates nerve and muscle function, and can lower blood pressure in people who have high blood pressure but not in those with normal blood pressure. Sources include green leafy vegetables, beans, nuts and seeds, many fruits and whole grains.

Selenium is an essential trace mineral. It acts as an antioxidant in much the same way as vitamin E. Only trace amounts are needed, but deficiencies have been linked with some birth defects and some first trimester miscarriages. Low levels of selenium have been found in some premature babies with respiratory problems and in mothers of babies with neural tube defects. Studies have shown that communities with high levels of selenium in the soil have low levels of cancer. Good sources of selenium include celery, garlic and onions, seafood, eggs, meat, whole grains, brazil nuts and broccoli.

Zinc is needed for strong bones and teeth, healthy hair and digestion, and is essential for the absorption of folic acid. Pregnant women often obtain only two-thirds of the recommended daily allowance of zinc. This has been associated with morning sickness, spina bifida, low birth weight and toxaemia of pregnancy. Zinc deficiency has also been implicated in the development of attention deficit disorder (ADD) as have low levels of essential fatty acids. Stretch marks indicate a need for zinc, and zinc supplementation may help to minimise them. Zinc levels decline significantly with advancing pregnancy. Males need zinc for the development of the genitals, the health of the prostate and for the manufacture of male hormones. Any skin problems such as dermatitis, acne or wounds that heal slowly often indicate a zinc deficiency. Good sources of zinc are whole grains, seafood, eggs, and sunflower and pumpkin seeds. Meat contains little or no zinc, so diets high in meat products may be zinc deficient.

WHAT SHOULD I EAT?

The following is a suggestion for a diet which will give you a wide variety of foods with a good range of nutrients and which will help you obtain the nutrients essential for a healthy pregnancy. Make sure that you use a variety of different foods from each category to ensure that you obtain a good balance of nutrients.

Table 2. Suggested Daily Diet

Category	Daily Servings	Foods
Green vegetables	3 serves - $^1/_2$ cup per serve	spinach, broccoli, celery, brussel sprouts, etc
Other vegetables	3 per day	pumpkin, carrot, cauliflower, zucchini, etc
Fruit	3 serves	one should be high in vitamin C (e.g. oranges)
Bread/cereals	6 - 11 serves - $^1/_2$ - 1 cup per serve	brown rice, oats, barley, buckwheat, millet (contains magnesium)

	1 slice of bread per serve	whole grain or wholemeal wheat or rye bread
Dairy	4 - 6 glasses	milk or equivalent in cheese and yoghurt
Protein	2 - 3 small serves	fish at least 2 - 3 times a week, meat, chicken, eggs, tofu, soy or other beans, nuts (e.g. almonds, cashews or brazil nuts) and seeds (e.g. sunflower, sesame or pumpkin)
Fats/oils	3 tsp - 3 Tbsp	olive oil, other cold pressed oils, mayonnaise, butter, etc
Water	8 - 10 glasses (1 - 2 litres)	filtered or spring water

If you have any allergies or food intolerances, you will need to adjust the diet. For example, if you are allergic to milk products, it will be very difficult for you to obtain your daily allowance for calcium from other sources and you will need to take a calcium supplement. If you are a vegetarian, you have special requirements. Please ensure that you obtain advice from an appropriately qualified practitioner.

Choose organic fruit and vegetables where possible. Always wash fruit and vegetables well. Buy free-range eggs and chickens.

Minimise the use of peanuts and peanut butter. Peanuts are susceptible to a fungus which produces toxic byproducts. They are also a highly allergic food. Use other nut butters – they are much tastier and much better for you.

Do not limit calories during pregnancy and lactation.

Drinks

Filtered water is preferable to tap water. You can add a little lemon or a small amount of fruit juice if you can't drink plain water. Herb teas, such as chamomile and peppermint, are refreshing and good for your digestion. Avoid coffee and caffeine containing drinks such as Coke. Don't drink decaffeinated coffee either – it has been processed with lots of chemicals. Tea is preferable to coffee if you must have either.

Snacks

Use fruit, yoghurt, nuts and seeds, wholemeal sandwiches, dips with vegetable crudites or baked potato as snacks. Minimise cakes, biscuits and other processed foods as they contain little nutrition and plenty of sugar and fat.

SOME CAUTIONS

Listeria

Avoid foods which may contain listeria. Listeria monocytogenes, commonly referred to as listeria, are bacteria which are spread by infected foods. While listeria is generally harmless to most people, it may cause serious symptoms in pregnancy, in individuals with a compromised immune system and in the elderly.

During pregnancy, the mother may experience no symptoms at all or may develop flu-like symptoms with fever, nausea and vomiting, headaches and generalised muscular aches and pains. Infection of the foetus may lead to meningitis, inflammation of the brain, or miscarriage. Newborn babies with listeriosis may develop chest infections and have breathing difficulties.

To reduce the risk of contracting listeriosis avoid the following: pate; soft and blue-veined cheeses; raw or unprocessed milk and milk products; pre-cooked meats such as ham; uncooked seafood; foods which have not been thoroughly cooked, particularly chicken; left-overs kept for more than two days; any foods which have not been freshly prepared, such as salads from delicatessens and salad bars; and leaving food at room temperature for any length of time.

Always wash fruit and vegetables carefully before use; store cooked and raw foods separately; thoroughly cook all meat, fish, eggs and poultry; completely heat through pre-cooked foods or meats such as hotdogs; and cover and refrigerate food.

Alcohol

Minimise or avoid the use of alcohol as the developing foetal brain seems to be particularly sensitive to the effects of alcohol damage. An occasional drink may be fine during pregnancy, but binge drinking has been associated with foetal abnormalities. Hyperactivity and short attention span have also been linked to alcohol use during pregnancy. The development of the entire central nervous system relies on adequate supplies of various nutrients. Alcohol use compromises the availability of these important nutrients to the foetus.

Foetal alcohol syndrome, FAS, is a serious condition which occurs in infants born to alcoholic mothers. Common problems associated with foetal alcohol syndrome include growth retardation, failure to thrive, feeding problems, persistent vomiting and mental retardation. Many of these children become hyperactive and experience learning difficulties.

Smoking

Smoking has been linked with an increased incidence of spontaneous abortion, preterm rupture of the membranes and low birth weight. Also more prevalent in smoking mothers are placental difficulties leading to bleeding, such as placenta previa, the attachment of the placenta to the lower part of the uterus, or abruptio placenta, and early detachment of the placenta before the due date. These risks are directly related to the number of cigarettes smoked, which means that the more you smoke, the greater the risk. It also seems that the longer you have smoked, the greater the risk to the baby.

Caffeine

Caffeine use has been linked to low birth weight. Sources of caffeine include coffee, cola drinks, tea and chocolate. Drink plenty of filtered water instead.

Chemicals

Many pesticides and radioactive substances are known to be harmful to the developing foetus. Many other substances are suspected, but conclusive data is lacking. In these circumstances, it is wise for the expectant mother to avoid chemicals wherever possible. Avoid using garden pesticides, heavy cleaning chemicals such as oven cleaners, and paints and solvents before as well as during pregnancy. The young baby should also be protected from such harmful substances while his immune system is developing.

Medication

Many medications are also known to be damaging to the growing foetus. Some vaccines are contraindicated. Over-the-counter drugs as well as prescription drugs may be contraindicated. For example, avoid aspirin as it may prolong labour and increase the risk of bleeding before labour. During the first trimester, the organs are developing so this is the most critical time for care with medication. Unfortunately, some women do not know they are pregnant until well into their first trimester and these women need to discuss with their doctor any use of medication before the pregnancy was confirmed. Some medications are necessary for certain conditions. Your doctor will prescribe one with the lowest known risk. If you are in any doubt about the use of a drug, consult your doctor.

Recreational Drugs

The effects of marijuana during pregnancy have been difficult to assess, possibly because of unreliable reporting of illegal substance use. Cocaine, however, has been shown to increase the risk of congenital abnormalities, premature birth, foetal distress and stillbirth.

WHAT IF I EAT WELL?

Studies have shown a decreased risk of birth defects, such as heart problems, in babies whose mothers took multivitamin supplements in the months preceding conception and throughout their pregnancies. Mothers with low levels of omega-3 fatty acids (found in linseed oil and fish oil) were found to have a greater risk of giving birth prematurely than mothers with high levels. Many studies have shown that we do not obtain sufficient amounts of zinc, iron, manganese and other nutrients from the average balanced diet. To get enough iron you would need to eat 700 – 800 g of spinach each day or 400 g of parsley. Liver and kidney are high in iron, but you would need to eat 200 – 500 g of either each day.

Doctors recognise the huge increase in nutritional needs during pregnancy and lactation, but they seem to concentrate on only three nutrients – calcium, iron and folic acid. Pregnant women are advised to increase their intake of these, but advice is rarely given on the importance of the other minerals and vitamins or the essential fatty acids.

As suggested in the detailed discussion on the various vitamins and minerals, the situation is quite complex and no one or two nutrients on their own can guarantee perfect health. It is always a matter of balance. So rather than relying on one or two nutrients, it is far more sensible to ensure that you have adequate levels of all known nutrients.

THE RECOMMENDED DAILY ALLOWANCE

There is some confusion about the values given for the recommended daily allowances (RDAs). It is important to keep in mind that RDA values have been determined as sufficient to avoid a frank deficiency state in healthy males in their early twenties eating an otherwise healthy diet. There are several problems associated with this way of setting RDAs:

- The values have been developed using a fit subgroup of the male population whose needs do not necessarily reflect the needs of other groups, particularly pregnant women.
- Their diet was otherwise healthy and did not include regular amounts of takeaway, processed or nutritionless food.
- The values for pregnancy have been extrapolated from these values, that is, they have been estimated from the available data. This may result in arbitrary figures.
- No recommendations can be made for people who are not healthy, who are not fit, who are over twenty years' old, and who are exposed to stress, pesticides, cigarette smoke and other pollutants.
- Daily requirements may be higher than the recommended values if there has been a continuous deficiency that has gone unnoticed.
- The RDAs are sufficient to just avoid a noticeable and immediate deficiency. No account has been taken of long-term health at these values or of long-term deficiencies.
- Research results showing improved health with doses higher than the RDA have not been used in the compilation of RDA values.
- Some of the recorded RDA levels have been questioned as dependent on the testing procedure and are therefore not an accurate measure of the true level. This is especially true for vitamin C. It has been suggested that the accepted RDA value for vitamin C has been assessed incorrectly and is far too low.

According to many studies our food does not contain the vitamins and minerals which we expect it to contain. Over the years we have depleted the soil of vital nutrients and have not replaced them. This has resulted in an ever increasing lack of nutrients in our foods.

This leads us to the conclusion that there are several difficulties associated with meeting our nutritional requirements. First, most of us rarely eat a well-balanced diet every day, but due to work and other commitments we often eat junk or processed food, with little nutritional value. For example, most women obtain only about seventy per cent of the RDA for thiamine, otherwise known as vitamin B1. These regular deficiencies increase our need for nutrients. Second, our food supply is deficient in the vitamins and minerals we need and so levels may be lower than suggested in guides to vitamin and mineral content of foods. Third, the RDAs are recognised to be too low, so we should aim for higher doses of all nutrients. Fourth, there is increasing evidence showing that supplementation with extra nutrients is beneficial to the health of both mother and baby.

SUPPLEMENTS RECOMMENDED IN PREGNANCY

In an ideal world we would obtain all our nutritional requirements from our food. Unfortunately, the world is not ideal and we are not always able to do this. To compensate for the lack in our food supply, supplementary vitamins and minerals may be necessary. We have already accepted the need for additional iron, calcium and folic acid during pregnancy, and the principles are the same for the other essential nutrients. Reasonable intakes of these nutrients guard against nutritional deficiencies which cause overt disease, such as spina bifida and osteoporosis. They also guard against low grade and not so spectacular deficiencies which nonetheless cause ill health and distress. To obtain a complete and balanced range of nutrients, the diet recommended in Table 2 is a good starting point. However, I also recommend that the supplements shown in Table 3 be taken every day:

Table 3. Recommendations for Supplements During Pregnancy

Note: Fat-soluble vitamins, such as vitamins A, D and E, require fats for their absorption. They are measured in international units (iu). Sometimes vitamin A may be measured in retinol equivalents (RE). One RE is roughly equivalent to 3.3 iu. 5000 iu is equal to 1500 RE is equal to 1.5 mg. Vitamin D, also referred to as cholecalciferol, may be measured in micrograms, with 1 mcg equal to 40 iu. Vitamin E may be measured in milligrams, with 1 mg equal to 1 iu.

Water-soluble vitamins are measured in milligrams (mg) and micrograms (mcg).

Vitamin A   2000 iu
        Vitamin A should be obtained from 3 mg beta carotene tablets.

A **multivitamin** containing

Vitamin B1 (thiamine)	50 mg
Vitamin B2 (riboflavin)	50 mg
Vitamin B3 (niacin)	50 mg
Vitamin B5 (pantothenate)	50 mg
Vitamin B6 (pyridoxine)	100 - 200 mg
Vitamin B12	100 mcg
Folic Acid	500 mcg
Vitamin D	400 iu
Vitamin E	400 – 500 iu
Vitamin K	500 mcg

A **multimineral** containing

Chromium	0.2 mg
Iron	20 mg

Manganese	10 mg
Molybdenum	100 mcg
Potassium	3 - 5g
Selenium	200 mcg
Zinc	20 mg

A **calcium and magnesium** supplement containing

Calcium	800 - 1200 mg
Magnesium	400 - 600 mg

The ideal calcium supplement contains magnesium, half as much as the amount of calcium. It also contains silica, which helps with the assimilation of calcium. The requirement for calcium is a total of 1200 mg each day. A serve of dairy food will give you about 250 mg of calcium, as will a standard supplement containing both calcium and magnesium. You need to calculate roughly how much you obtain from your diet and then calculate the amount you need to obtain from your supplement. You will obtain some calcium and magnesium from meat, fish, nuts and seeds, and small amounts of these minerals may also be in your multimineral supplement. If you cannot tolerate dairy foods, plan to obtain a good proportion of your calcium requirement from your supplement.

An **essential fatty acid** supplement

Evening primrose oil and fish oil supplement – 1000 mg 1 - 3 times a day or 1 - 2 tablespoons of linseed oil

Take the higher value if there is any family history of allergy, asthma, skin disorders or attention deficit disorder.

Vitamin C   1000 - 2000 mg

Take the higher value if you get frequent colds.

Probiotics

Acidophilus and bifidus   1 - 2 tablets daily, up to
                                   2 tablets three times a
                                   day if there is candida
                                   or thrush

After the second trimester, to prepare the uterus, add

Raspberry leaf tea or tablets   one tablet or one cup
                                    three times a day

You may also consider visiting a naturopath to obtain a balancing herbal supplement. The herbs generally recommended
have a long history of use before and during pregnancy to prepare the uterus for childbirth, to avoid premature labour and
to reduce false labour pains.

These recommendations are for healthy women. Some
women will have special needs and these should be super-
vised by a health practitioner. If you can answer yes to any of
the following questions, you may have special needs:

- Have you given birth less than two years before your cur-
  rent pregnancy?
- Do you have allergies or a family history of allergy?
- Have you miscarried in the past?
- Are you expecting twins?
- Have you been on the Pill?
- Have you ever been seriously ill or had major surgery?
- Do you smoke or work with chemicals? You should not
  smoke during pregnancy, but the sad fact is that some
  women continue to do so regardless of the overwhelming
  evidence that smoking is harmful to the unborn child.
  These mothers need to be extra careful and need special
  advice.
- Are you a vegetarian?

If you are concerned about your requirements, visit a naturopath or nutritional therapist to discuss your needs. There are special supplements designed especially for use during pregnancy. A practitioner will also check that your diet is adequate and that your nutritional intake is balanced.

Chapter 3

HERBS

Herbs have been used by many communities to treat most common health complaints. Every country has its tradition of herbal use; indeed, herbs were the first form of medicine before the advent of antibiotics and other pharmaceuticals. Uses for the herbs were learnt by the women of the community, who provided the earliest health care.

Many countries still rely heavily on the medicinal properties of herbs. In Europe many medical practitioners regularly prescribe herbs for many common complaints. Herbs must satisfy the same legal requirements as any other drug in terms of safety and efficacy. The wide use of herbs in many European countries has ensured that they are monitored regularly for quality and safety. China has a strong tradition of herbal medicine and many of the Chinese herbs are now available in other countries. India has its Ayurvedic medicine, which uses herbs and diet to maintain and encourage good health. Other parts of Asia have their own traditions of herbal medicines. In America herbs are less easily available as legal restrictions make it difficult for suppliers to make any claims about the efficacy of their product. Similarly, in Australia, there are restrictions on disseminating information about herbs. Despite these restrictions, consumers in America and Australia are recognising the role of herbs in their health care and there are now many practitioners recommending and supplying herbs. Some Australian universities are researching the uses and safety of herbs and there are postgraduate studies for nurses and medical practitioners in the uses of herbs.

Many pharmaceutical drugs have been extracted from plants. For example, digitalis, a herb traditionally used for heart disorders, has given us digoxin, the pharmaceutical drug used in heart failure. The analgesics codeine and morphine are derived from opium and the poppy plant. Aspirin is a member of the salicylate family, which was originally extracted from willow bark. These pharmaceutical uses have been derived from, and have supported, the traditional uses of the original herbs. Native plants from various countries are currently being studied for their healing effects. Extracts of some of these plants or synthetic copies of their active ingredients will go on to be developed as new pharmaceutical drugs.

Herbalists believe that the body has an inherent wisdom and power of self-healing. Herbs can encourage this tendency towards health and harmony in the body. Herbalists also believe that herbs are balanced, that is, that any herb is 'greater than the sum of its parts' and that extracting and refining single ingredients from plant material disregards many important synergistic effects of the whole plant. A typical example of this can be noted in the use of the dandelion herb or celery as diuretics to encourage fluid loss through more frequent urination. Both these herbs contain potassium, which is often leached by frequent urination. Therefore, the appreciable amounts of potassium offset the potential problem of excessive potassium loss.

Improvements in the extraction of herbs have led to the standardisation of their active ingredients. This allows for more accurate prescribing and guarantees quality control and a standard, defined level of potency of the herb product. With improvements in technology, herbs can be identified accurately, harvested at the optimum times to maximise active ingredients, stored in ideal conditions for plant stability and checked for impurities. All this further guarantees the safety and efficacy of the final product.

The herbs described here have been recommended for use in pregnancy, labour, during lactation or for the baby for the conditions described in the relevant chapters. The following discussion of the herbs gives a brief description of each and some of their common uses as well as some information about their specific use during pregnancy, labour and the post-partum period. When using herbal products do not ever exceed the recommended dosage and use them only for the time necessary for the ailment or complaint to be resolved. If you are in any doubt about the use or dosage of a herb, consult a naturopath or herbalist.

The most commonly used herbs during pregnancy are the uterine tonics or partus preparators used to tone and prepare the uterus for labour. These include black haw, blue cohosh, cramp bark, false unicorn root, red raspberry leaf and squaw vine.

These partus preparators tone the uterine muscle and often improve blood supply to the pelvic area. They promote regular, coordinated and effective contractions during labour. They encourage greater comfort for the mother as the uterus is allowed to relax fully between contractions. These effects are particularly useful if a long labour leads to fatigue and loss of uterine tone. These herbs also have a reputation for calming and soothing the nervous system, allowing the labouring mother to remain calm and focussed.

The same herbs have the opposite effect during pregnancy. The effect is relaxing during pregnancy as the antispasmodic and calming properties reduce uterine irritability, thus decreasing the risk of premature labour. This calming effect reduces spasms and Braxton Hicks contractions.

These partus preparators should be taken during the third trimester to benefit from both the calming and toning effects. They can also be used during labour to maintain strong, regular and coordinated contractions while allowing the uterus to rest between contractions.

Black Haw (Viburnum Prunifolium)

Black haw is a uterine tonic and partus preparator.

Blessed Thistle

Blessed thistle, also known as Holy thistle, has toning effects on the digestive system, increasing the flow of bile and stimulating the liver. Its best-known use is to increase milk production.

Calendula

Calendula is soothing to the digestive system, reducing inflammation which may lead to indigestion and pain after eating. As a topical preparation, it has strong antiseptic and wound-healing properties. This makes calendula useful in nipple care, nappy rash, care of the umbilical cord or for any cuts, insect bites or abrasions.

Blue Cohosh (Caulophyllum)

Blue cohosh is a uterine tonic used frequently in preparation for labour and childbirth.

Chamomile

Chamomile flowers are widely used both internally and externally. Internally, chamomile tea is taken to soothe an inflamed digestive system. It is very relaxing for the digestive system, reducing tension, spasms and pain. This makes it useful for many of the digestive upsets of babies and young children. It reduces spasms, inflammation and nausea, colic and wind, and also the growth of harmful bacteria and fungi. Chamomile tea, with its soothing and calming properties, is often useful in the nausea of pregnancy. It is especially effective if the discomfort is caused by nervous tension, such as when stressed or eating in a hurry.

Always prepare your own tea from the flowers, as many chamomile tea bags do not contain sufficient amounts of the active ingredients.

Painful conditions such as headache, arthritis, and painful joints or muscles often respond to massage with the essential oil or to a relaxing bath infused with chamomile. Externally, infusions of the flowers or preparations of essential oil are used for any skin inflammation, including eczema, nappy rash and cradle cap.

Cramp Bark (Viburnum Opulus)

Cramp bark is another uterine tonic.

Dandelion Root and Herb

Dandelion, otherwise known as Taraxacum officinale, has been used widely in Europe for the treatment of various liver and kidney complaints. There are two preparations of dandelion, the root and the herb or leaf. Dandelion leaf or herb has a strong diuretic effect on the kidneys. It promotes urination, making it very useful for relieving fluid retention. Dandelion herb is also useful if there is any mild infection in the urinary tract.

The root of the plant has a tonic effect, predominantly on the liver, and is used to stimulate digestion if there is indigestion or loss of appetite. It has a mild laxative effect and may relieve some cases of nausea. Dandelion root is used in China for many breast problems, such as inflammation, mastitis and reduced milk flow.

Echinacea

Echinacea is a widely used herb, with a long history of use by the native Americans. Relying on echinacea's properties as an immune system stimulant, the American Indians used it to treat serious viral and bacterial infections, snakebite and wounds. Interest in echinacea spread to Europe, where it has been extensively researched, most recently by the European Scientific Cooperative on Phytotherapy (ESCOP). There are three commonly used species of echinacea: echinacea angustifolia, echinacea purpurea and echinacea pallida. They are often combined to utilise the differing concentrations of the active ingredients in each of the species. The root of the plant contains the greatest concentration of active ingredients and is more effective in very acute complaints, but the whole herb can be used as a preventative or in mild conditions.

European doctors prescribe echinacea regularly. Numerous studies have found no evidence of any danger in its use during pregnancy. As with any preparation – herbal, food or pharmaceutical – allergic reactions are possible, but with echinacea, these occur only occasionally in intravenous usage or in those with extreme allergic sensitivities.

Echinacea has received a great deal of bad press in Australia and it has been suggested that it may cause asthmatic attacks or even anaphylactic shock leading to death in susceptible individuals. These reactions have not been supported by overseas studies, nor have the proponents of these warnings been able to produce any direct evidence for their claims. The purported reasons for problems associated with echinacea use have not been supported by experimental evidence or population-based studies. Several prominent Australian doctors who are leaders in their fields of integrative and nutritional medicine have refuted these claims about the dangers of echinacea and noted the irresponsibility of claims which have not been able to be scientifically verified. They point out that, given the huge doses of echinacea consumed annually by Australians, it is a very safe and important herb in the treatment of immune disorders, including asthma.

Echinacea is used whenever there is any infection anywhere in the body. It is frequently used for colds or flu, but it can be effective for any type of infection, such as skin abscess or boils, chest infections, ear and throat infections, mastitis and candida. Echinacea is very effective when used to prevent colds and flu during peak seasons or for susceptible individuals. If you are using echinacea for prevention, a less potent preparation is recommended than if you are using it during an acute attack.

False Unicorn Root

False unicorn root has a reputation as a uterine tonic and has been used to prevent threatened miscarriage and haemorrhage. It is also used to improve female fertility as it has a normalising effect on ovarian function during the menstrual cycle.

Fennel

Fennel is often used as a culinary herb. It supports the digestive system by promoting digestive enzymes. It is very calming for the digestive system, relaxing spasms and colic. Fennel can be used as a tea or the essential oil may be used in a massage blend. Fennel oil is an ingredient in Gripe Water, which is used to relieve infant colic.

Garlic

Garlic is a herb used commonly in cooking, but it is also known for its antibacterial, antiviral, antifungal and antimicrobial properties. Preparations of garlic can inhibit many bacteria and viruses, including those which cause many throat infections, coughs, colds, runny noses, hay fever, and sinus and chest infections. Candida, which causes thrush, can often be controlled successfully with the addition of garlic to your medical treatment.

Include some garlic in your diet regularly. If you do not want to or cannot use garlic regularly for social reasons, there are some odourless preparations of garlic available that do not cause the same social embarrassment as fresh garlic. While some people are sensitive to garlic and feel that it repeats on them, most are fine with some of the better quality odourless garlic preparations.

Garlic is also being used to lower blood pressure, high cholesterol and raised triglycerides.

Ginger

Ginger stimulates the digestive system and encourages digestive enzymes to act on food. It also settles and calms the stomach by relaxing and reducing spasms. These effects will often reduce nausea and indigestion. This makes ginger valuable for many cases of nausea during pregnancy, for post-operative vomiting and for travel sickness. Grated fresh ginger can be taken regularly; alternatively, there are ginger tablets which are perhaps more convenient.

Ginger also has anti-inflammatory properties and is an ingredient in many preparations for arthritis and migraine headaches.

Hamamelis (Witch-hazel)

Used topically, witch-hazel soothes swelling or burning of the skin from minor cuts, insect bites or abrasions. It quickly stops any associated bleeding and protects against infection. Applied to varicose veins or haemorrhoids, it reduces the pain, itching and swelling. It helps maintain the integrity of the blood vessel wall, preventing and, in some people, even reversing many of the symptoms of haemorrhoids.

Hops

Hops reduce tension and spasms in the body, encouraging deep and restful sleep. This effect is most noticeable where there is muscle tension in the body or if there are spasms in the digestive system. Lack of sleep resulting from tension, stress or anxiety may respond to the calming properties of hops. By soothing the digestive system, hops encourage improved digestion and may be used whenever stress and anxiety affect the digestion.

Hops are a major ingredient in beer and may partly explain the relaxing effect of beer at the end of a long, hard day. Only one or two glasses are needed for the calming and relaxing effects. Taken to excess the effect is often just the opposite, demonstrating the well-known adage that 'more is not necessarily better'.

Horse Chestnut

Horse chestnut, like witch-hazel, is used for problems with the veins. Pain and swelling from varicose veins or haemorrhoids often respond to the use of horse chestnut. It is usually given as a herb rather than as a topical preparation. Horse chestnut is an ingredient in many herbal preparations for the circulatory system because of its powerful effect in strengthening blood vessel walls.

Linseed

Linseed contains essential fatty acids, which may help in the treatment of skin disorders such as dryness, eczema and psoriasis. It is a good source of easily digestible protein, many important minerals and vitamins A and E. Linseed contains fibre and is useful in constipation or where there is any irritability or inflammation of the intestines. It acts as a laxative and stabilises blood sugar levels.

Linseed has a very hard outer coat which is not easily broken by the human digestive system. Use linseed ground into a fine powder. Freshly ground linseed is best as the oils in linseed oxidise quickly when exposed to the air. If you are not able to grind your own seeds, purchase ground seeds in a sealed packet and refrigerate them in a sealed container. Use within two weeks of opening. Always drink plenty of water with the linseed as it absorbs moisture from your digestive system.

Linseed oil, often called flax oil, is also available and is a rich source of the essential fatty acids necessary for healthy skin. Use edible flax oil, not linseed oil bought at the hardware store, as this is not for internal use.

Melissa (Lemon Balm)

Melissa is very calming for the digestive system. It may be effective for nausea, vomiting, colic and especially if there is any anxiety or nervousness affecting the digestion. With its calming and soothing properties, melissa has been used for headaches including migraine, for anxiety and depression.

Peppermint

Peppermint is very refreshing, and has a relaxing and calming effect. Taken as a tea, it relaxes the muscles of the digestive system and reduces spasms and indigestion. It is very effective for many cases of nausea, heartburn, stomach-ache and vomiting. Peppermint protects the lining of the digestive system, reducing irritation and colic. Peppermint oil is one of the ingredients of Gripe Water. It is also recommended for irritable bowel syndrome, a condition with spasm, flatulence and pain in the intestines, often accompanied by alternating bouts of diarrhoea and constipation.

Passionflower Herb

Passionflower is a very relaxing and calming herb. Reducing spasms and tension in the muscles and calming the nervous system, it is a useful herb whenever there is any stress, anxiety, tension, mood changes, nervousness or restlessness. It is often used for sleeplessness due to stress, anxiety or overwork.

Psyllium

Psyllium (pronounced syllium, the 'p' is silent) is the seed and husk of the plant ispaghula or plantago. It has a very high fibre content. The husks and seeds are ground into a meal. Used predominantly as a laxative, psyllium is also effective in diarrhoea, making it very useful in the treatment of irritable bowel syndrome. It protects the lining of the intestines by inhibiting the attachment of toxic compounds, including bacteria. It also lowers cholesterol.

Psyllium is very useful during pregnancy as a laxative and for its soothing effect on the digestive system.

Red Raspberry Leaves

Raspberry leaves are best known for their toning effect on the uterus in preparation for childbirth and for helping recovery and involution of the uterus after the birth. Raspberry leaves also help with milk production for the nursing mother.

Squaw Vine (Partridge Berry, Mitchella Repens)

As the name suggests, this is a North American Indian herb used to tone and strengthen the uterus in preparation for childbirth.

St John's Wort

Also known as hypericum, St John's wort is used in any state of tension, stress, anxiety or depression. Sleeplessness associated with these states responds well to the use of St John's wort. It has been used for centuries in Europe for its antidepressant activity and studies have compared it favourably to Prozac. For this reason, it has been called the 'herbal Prozac'. Unlike Prozac, it has few side effects.

During and after pregnancy it has many possible uses. Stress and anxiety during pregnancy prevent you from enjoying your pregnancy. St John's wort may be helpful in this case. Postnatal depression may also respond to its use. In cases of serious and long-lasting depression, always seek professional advice and counselling to uncover the reason for your state of mind. St John's wort, however, may be a useful addition to your treatment protocol.

St John's wort is also effective against certain viruses, including those that cause herpes. This includes both types of herpes. Herpes simplex 1 causes cold sores, so regular sufferers should take St John's wort regularly as a preventative measure. Outbreaks of herpes simplex 2, which causes genital herpes, may also be controlled with regular use of the herb. St John's wort has also been used successfully against the Epstein Barr virus, which causes glandular fever. Studies are also confirming its benefits in treating HIV/AIDS.

Externally, the oil of St John's wort can be used on blunt injuries or wherever there is sharp pain.

Valerian

Valerian is an important herb for the relief of anxiety and sleeplessness. It has a strong sedative effect, encouraging sleep, reducing night time waking and improving the quality of sleep. It does not cause daytime sleepiness or difficulties in concentrating; in fact, it can aid concentration as its anti-anxiety properties help you to focus on one thing at a time.

Occasionally some people find that valerian does not

improve their sleep, in which case use another herb such as hops or passionflower. Reducing the dosage helps if you still feel a little foggy in the morning. If you have had a long period of sleeplessness, it may take a while for you to recover fully from the effects of stress and missed sleep. In this case, it may not be the fault of the valerian if you feel foggy in the morning; it may be that your body is still tired and the valerian is helping you to relax.

Vitex Agnus Castus (Agnus Castus or Chaste Tree)

Vitex agnus castus stimulates milk production. It is best known for its balancing effect on the female hormone progesterone. This hormone acts predominantly during the second half of the female menstrual cycle and is often out of balance if there is premenstrual syndrome (PMS). This makes vitex agnus castus useful for heavy or painful periods, mood swings and weepiness prior to menstruation. It is balancing after use of the contraceptive pill.

Chapter 4

AROMATHERAPY AND ESSENTIAL OILS

Pregnancy is a time to look after yourself well and to spoil yourself. Aromatherapy uses essential oils which, with their wonderful rich smells, provide a beautiful way to pamper as well as care for yourself safely. Essential oils are becoming widely used in all aspects of health care. Many nurses are being trained in their use and are incorporating them into their patient care. Many labour wards encourage the use of oils as their benefits are becoming more understood and appreciated.

Aromatherapy literally means treatment using aromatic substances. These aromatic substances are called essential oils. They are prepared from plants and are highly concentrated. Many are made from the flowers of the plant, but they may also be prepared from the bark of a tree, from the fruit or the seeds.

As the oil is extracted from the plant, it concentrates the plant's properties, giving a powerful essence with the therapeutic and healing powers of the original plant. Essential oils have a clean, healthy and fresh smell. They contain a vast array of ingredients, far too many to be produced synthetically. For this reason choose essential oils rather than fragrant oils. Fragrant oils are man-made and do not have the therapeutic properties of essential oils. Fragrant oils are much cheaper than essential oils, but often smell very sweet and cloying.

Some oils require a lot of the original plant to obtain only small amounts of oil; therefore, these oils may be very expensive. Jasmine, neroli and rose oils are in this category.

The properties of essential oils include antiseptic, anti-inflammatory, anti-fungal, relaxing, uplifting or stimulating actions. Many are balancing or normalising and most have a range of actions, which means that they can be used for a variety of purposes.

Their effects are achieved in two ways. The first effect involves the connection of our nostrils to our limbic system, a part of the brain concerned with emotions. Components of the essential oils are transmitted to our limbic system when the oil vapours are in the air we breathe. They can affect our feelings of sadness or depression, helping us to feel calmer, more relaxed and less anxious. Some oils, such as neroli and clary sage, have quite strong positive effects on our emotions. This effect has been verified even in situations when we cannot smell the oil, such as when we have a head cold or when we have become accustomed to the aroma. Very small amounts of oil are needed to achieve this effect.

The second effect of essential oils involves their affinity with particular body organs. For example, tea tree oil has a strong effect on the respiratory system and can be used whenever anyone in the house has a cold. Rose oil tones and strengthens the digestive and circulatory systems. Chamomile oil has anti-inflammatory properties and can be used whenever there is pain or swelling. Generally essential oils have a number of healing properties and benefit a number of body systems. Most oils are of benefit to both our emotional and physical health.

To achieve these benefits, the oils can be used in a number of ways. The various methods of use will be discussed fully later in this chapter. Briefly, however, oils can be used to permeate the air, or they can be applied directly for absorption by the skin via a massage or in a bath. We use chest rubs during a cold, giving the benefits of both smell and direct application to the area. We apply massage blends to sore, tight muscle areas to direct the healing properties quickly to the area in need. Surprisingly, however, the essential oil does not always need to be applied directly to the affected area. The oil will diffuse into the bloodstream and travel to the area where it is needed. This is especially true when the oil benefits internal organs. Remember, however, that essential oils, with their rich array of components, will demonstrate a number of healing properties, and their mode of use in any circumstance depends on personal preference, convenience and other considerations.

Some essential oils are especially recommended during pregnancy, while others are contraindicated. A list of these recommended essential oils and their uses follows. The recommended oils are perfectly safe if used in a massage blend, in a burner or a vaporiser. Never take essential oils by mouth.

You will need only a couple of drops of essential oil at any time, so although oils seem expensive, they will last a long time and are good value for money. Keep them stored in a dark cupboard and mix them only as you need them. If you collect a number of oils, there are attractive wooden boxes specially designed to store them safely.

OILS TO USE DURING PREGNANCY AND LABOUR

Essential oils can be used safely during pregnancy to encourage a peaceful and relaxed feeling, to aid restful sleep, to provide antibacterial and antiviral actions, or to provide a homely and comforting atmosphere. They can also be used during labour to help calm and relax you. Along with other techniques used for pain relief, use your oils to soothe anxiety and feelings of panic. Women who have used essential oils regularly during their pregnancy seem to obtain the most benefit from their use during labour. Their bodies are aware of the oil's nurturing properties and respond to them more quickly and easily. However, even if you have not used oils during your pregnancy, you will still benefit from their use during labour.

Chamomile

There are two types of chamomile – German, or blue chamomile, and Roman chamomile. Both are anti-inflammatory, which means that they will soothe any inflammation in the skin or the muscles. Chamomile soothes frayed nerves, aids sleep and relaxation, and is great for muscular aches and pains.

It is a relatively expensive oil and is used by professional massage therapists and aromatherapists. You can buy mixtures with two per cent chamomile in jojoba oil quite cheaply, but these do not have the same therapeutic value as the concentrated essential oil. Mixtures with jojoba oil should not be used in a burner as the jojoba oil may sputter when heated.

Eucalyptus

With its strong antiseptic effect on the respiratory system, eucalyptus is a good oil to have around the room whenever colds and flu are prevalent. Just a few drops in a burner, on a cotton ball or in a vaporiser will cleanse the air of germs and can help prevent flu spreading through the family. It is also good for muscular aches and pains, but you need only a drop in a massage blend or burner as it is a very strong smelling oil.

Geranium

A very light floral oil, geranium is refreshing and relaxing. It is both sedative and uplifting, and is often used for the relief of anxiety. As it has astringent properties, it has been used to help prevent haemorrhoids and varicose veins. It has been used postnatally for breast engorgement and in massage blends to increase milk flow.

Lavender

Lavender is a great all-purpose oil. Most people like the smell of lavender and it is safe for everyone, including newborn babies. It is one of the very few oils mild enough to be used straight on adult skin. It is good for the skin as it aids in healing and is recommended after burns and bites. It also helps to speed up the recovery of perineal wounds. It is very relaxing, has antidepressant qualities and is useful for relieving muscular aches and pains. Early in labour, a bath containing lavender has been found to be relaxing and nurturing.

Lavender is also one of the least expensive oils. Whether you intend to buy only one oil or would like to start a collection, I recommend lavender as your first purchase.

Neroli

This is a very expensive oil, but is one of the most relaxing, calming oils available. Neroli is one of the ingredients of eau-de-cologne as it has a beautiful aroma. It may be used throughout pregnancy, during labour and postnatally, to calm and relieve stress and to dispel any tension or anxiety.

Petitgrain

Called the 'poor man's neroli', petitgrain is a light, pleasant oil with properties similar to neroli. Therefore, it can be used whenever you need a little emotional lift or relaxation.

Rose

Rose has a strong affinity for the reproductive system with a toning and cleansing effect on the uterus. It is calming and soothing, encouraging deep breathing, and has strong antidepressant properties. For these reasons rose essential oil is highly recommended during labour. It is strongly antiseptic and has been used in the treatment of jaundice. It is a very expensive oil, but is available in some blends. Use rose oil in the bath or in massage blends.

Sandalwood

Sandalwood is a deep, woody oil that is very soothing and calming. It is a good oil to use whenever there is stress or anxiety. Use sandalwood in a burner, in a bath or a massage blend. It calms the digestive and respiratory systems.

Tangerine

Tangerine oil is a member of the citrus family. It is a light, mild oil. It is uplifting, but also calming and relaxing. It helps the skin to stretch, reducing the incidence of stretch marks. Tangerine is useful in a blend which you could rub into your growing tummy.

Ylang Ylang

A very pleasant, calming and relaxing oil, ylang ylang is used for any anxious or worried state. It is very useful during pregnancy and labour. It also has a reputation as an aphrodisiac and is often included in romantic blends. It is very soothing to the skin.

WAYS TO USE ESSENTIAL OILS

Massage

Have a massage as often as you can. If you have never had a massage before, this is definitely the time to start. Massage is very nurturing and soothing. Massage during pregnancy is generally much more gentle than at other times and will relax you as well as add moisture to your skin. You will find that you sleep very well after a relaxing massage. In fact, some of my clients claim that the only time they have a decent night's sleep is after their massage. The massage blend will contain moisturising oils to help your skin to stretch.

When you visit a massage therapist you will be asked a number of questions about your general health and whether there are any particular problems you would like to have addressed. If you are at all nervous, mention this at the start of the visit. Perhaps initially book just a half-hour massage. As you become more comfortable with your therapist, you will find that you relax more easily and may wish to consider a full-hour long massage.

After your massage, relax for a short time before driving home. Plan to go straight home rather than to the shops or visiting. This will give you the opportunity to relax and savour the effects and full benefits of your massage. Do not wash the oils off straight away. Allow them to remain on your skin as they will be absorbed slowly over the next few hours.

Massage at Home

You and your partner can learn some simple but effective massage techniques. Massage is a very loving and caring way to help and support each other. We often massage instinctively, but if you prefer some training, there are many short courses and books available to guide you through the basics.

Massage Blends

You need a carrier oil to which you add a couple of drops of your chosen essential oil. The carrier oil allows the massage therapist's hands to glide smoothly over the skin. It acts as a carrier for the essential oil you choose, and it moistens and nourishes the skin. Always choose cold pressed vegetable oils. These oils are absorbed by the skin and provide vitamins essential for healthy skin. Mineral-based oils such as baby oil act as a barrier, clog the pores and do not supply vitamins to the skin. Choose from the following:

- Almond oil is a good light oil which suits all skin types. It blends with most oils as it has no strong smell of its own. It can be used on babies.
- Grapeseed oil is another light oil. It is easily available and does not have a strong smell.
- Jojoba oil is a very moisturising oil which is easily absorbed by the skin and is suitable for all skin types. It can also be used on babies.

For a massage blend you will need about 30 ml of your carrier oil and two drops of your essential oil. You might choose to use only one essential oil in your blend. If you would like to use more than one, add no more than two or three different essential oils to your carrier oil. Mix only as much oil as you need to use at any one time because the essential oils evaporate fairly quickly and you will not receive the full benefits if the blend sits around for a while.

Baths and Foot Baths

A warm bath is another wonderful way to relax and revitalise. Play some relaxing music, Baroque or New Age music or any personal favourites. Have the bath warm, but not hot. Add about five drops of one or two of your favourite oils. Mix them well into the water before you enter the bath. Plan to go straight to bed afterwards. You will sleep deeply and wake feeling very refreshed.

If you do not have time for a full bath, you will experience similar relaxing benefits if you soak your feet for about fifteen to twenty minutes in a warm foot bath to which you have added a few drops of essential oil. There are some great foot spas available, which swirl the water and massage your feet, but a bucket will also do very nicely. Try to get one in which you can stretch out your feet, either a large round bowl or a rectangular bucket.

Burners and Vaporisers

A room filled with the aroma of your favourite essential oil is a nurturing and welcoming place. This is easy to achieve if you have a burner or a vaporiser. Use your oils at any time during the day or night to create a relaxing atmosphere or to keep the room smelling fresh and healthy. You can also use essential oils if anyone in the home has a cold or the flu.

There are some beautiful burners available, nowadays they are often works of art. To use your burner correctly you need to do the following:

- The well at the top must be filled with water.
- Light a candle in the lower part of the burner. Candles for burners are easily available in the right size. Choose the

more expensive candles as these do not burn as hot as the cheaper ones, so your precious oils will not evaporate so quickly, nor will your water dry up in the well as quickly.

- Add a couple of drops of an essential oil. You can add a couple of different oils, but do not use more than three at a time as the odours become a bit confused and I believe you confuse the body a little, too.
- Regularly top up the water – your burner will crack if the well dries out.
- Do not leave a burner unattended. If you have small children, keep the burner well out of their reach and ensure that you are always in the room. If you leave the house, blow out the candle.
- Do not have your candle alight at night.
- Do not use a candle near a curtain which might catch against the flame.

There are some electric burners available which do not become as hot as the ones with a candle. These, too, should be filled with water, but it is not so critical to regularly check the water level. As there is no naked flame, they are safer to use, especially around young children.

If you have a vaporiser, follow the manufacturer's instructions. This generally involves adding a couple of drops of oil to the water in the well at the top. Do not put essential oil into the main body of the vaporiser.

The effect of using a burner or vaporiser is well worth the effort involved. The aroma of the evaporating oils will fill the air and you will experience the healing benefits of whatever oils you have chosen. After a while you will become accustomed to the smell, but don't be tempted to top up the oil immediately. Leave the room for a while and you will smell the oil again when you return. Add more oil if the aroma has gone completely. More expensive brands will generally last longer than cheaper brands. Deeper, woody oils such as sandalwood will also last longer than floral, light oils such as geranium.

If you cannot use a burner because you have young children or for any other reason, you can still experience the benefits of essential oils by putting a few drops on a cotton ball or in a saucer of warm water. This is a safe way to have oils in the bedrooms, especially at night. A few drops of lavender by the bed encourages deeper, more restful sleep.

Chapter 5

SOME COMMON COMPLAINTS
OF PREGNANCY

There are a number of complaints which frequently plague pregnant women. Many of these are regarded as an inevitable part of pregnancy. Others are considered to be minor problems and generally they are not serious or dangerous except in certain circumstances. However, they can still prevent you from enjoying your pregnancy. Fortunately, many of them can be relieved effectively and safely using some simple measures. Anything that contributes to your wellbeing and comfort during pregnancy will help you to enjoy both your pregnancy and motherhood. Severe and serious problems must always be discussed with your doctor.

The measures suggested here include herbal remedies, homoeopathic remedies, Bach flower remedies, and vitamins and minerals. Therapies such as Bowen therapy, massage, osteopathic treatment and acupuncture may also be helpful and used safely. If your complaint persists in spite of these measures, discuss it with your doctor. If he or she is satisfied that there is no serious underlying condition, consider consulting a naturopath, herbalist or homoeopath for further advice. (See chapter 11 for a description of the various therapies and contacts for further information.)

Backache and Groin Pain

Backache during pregnancy is not an inevitability. Massage, Bowen therapy and gentle osteopathic treatment may be effective in relieving backache. Gentle exercise such as water aerobics and yoga helps to strengthen the back and relieve backache. Make sure that your bed supports your back adequately. If you need to lift other children, always bend your knees and stand next to something on which you can lean. Where possible, sit and then lift the child onto your lap.

Bowen therapy is particularly effective for the groin pain characteristic of relaxing joints and ligaments in late pregnancy. Gentle osteopathic treatment may also be effective for some back pain.

Braxton Hicks Contractions

Braxton Hicks contractions are often painful and powerful contractions which occur during the last few weeks of pregnancy. They may be regular and last for several hours. They can be annoying at best or totally disruptive at worst, and may sometimes be interpreted as true labour. Unlike true labour, however, they eventually fade with time. They prepare the cervix before labour and may even generate some dilation before true labour begins.

Frequent rest, preferably lying on the side rather than the back, is vital to avoid exhaustion. There are several herbs which can help the uterus to relax during pregnancy and which have a reputation for decreasing the risk of premature labour. In their capacity as relaxants they can diminish the discomfort experienced during Braxton Hicks contractions. The herbs needed here include squaw vine, false unicorn root, black haw and cramp bark. You may need to see a practitioner for these herbs and for correct dosage.

The tissue salts Calc Phos and Mag Phos can also help. Both of these are indicated whenever there is cramping or any type of spasm. Chew one of each three times a day if you are experiencing frequent Braxton Hicks contractions, or chew one of each every twenty to thirty minutes whenever the contractions start. These tissue salts will not affect the contractions if true labour has started, but will make you feel more comfortable with them.

Carpal Tunnel Syndrome

Bowen therapy is most effective for carpal tunnel syndrome, which involves pain and inflammation of the wrist resulting from pressure on the nerve. It often causes pain in the hand and forearm. Usually only one or two treatments are required to keep the pain down until your baby is born. The problem usually resolves after the birth. If it persists after the birth you may need surgery, but continue with a few more Bowen treatments and you may be able to avoid this.

Vitamin B6 is effective for some carpal tunnel syndrome sufferers. If you are already taking a multi-B supplement, include an extra 50 - 100 mg of vitamin B6 daily for a few days. You may also need extra magnesium, so take the tissue salt Mag Phos, one tablet four times a day.

Colds and Flu

Antibiotic use is generally discouraged, where possible, during pregnancy. There are other things you could try first if your cold or flu is not serious enough to warrant considering antibiotics. Prevention is always better than cure. Daily vitamin C or echinacea can be used to minimise your risk of catching infections. To help prevent the spread of flu germs, have a drop of eucalyptus oil in a burner or vaporiser around the house.

However, if you do catch a cold or the flu, there are some safe preparations you can use. Echinacea is a powerful immune system stimulant and has been used frequently during infection of the respiratory tract and lower urinary tract. Echinacea is safe to use during pregnancy and is readily available. Follow the dosage on the bottle. This dosage will depend on the strength of the brand you have chosen. The cost of the preparation will generally reflect the strength. The root is the strongest part of the plant and is the best part to use while battling a virus; however, the less expensive herb is fine as a preventative measure.

Garlic is also safe during pregnancy and lactation. It is antibacterial and can be used for coughs, colds, sinus infections and runny nose. Use one of the odourless preparations in the recommended dosage.

The tissue salt Ferrum Phos is useful when the cold starts. Take or chew a tablet frequently during the day. If there is any white mucous from the nose, also chew a Kali Mur tablet. If the mucous becomes yellow in colour, indicating a more serious infection, use Calc Sulph instead of the Kali Mur.

Alternatively, you might use an over-the-counter homoeopathic cold and flu preparation to overcome the virus.

Constipation (see also haemorrhoids)

Plenty of fibre in the form of fresh fruit and vegetables and high-fibre cereals, daily exercise such as walking, and plenty of fresh water will resolve most constipation problems. If you are still constipated, you can increase your fibre intake. Wheat bran is not always the best form of fibre; try oat bran, ground linseed or psyllium. Always increase your fibre slowly – start with one teaspoon and increase over the next few days if necessary.

If your iron supplement is causing constipation, try another brand. The constipation suggests that you may not be absorbing your supplement properly. Your iron supplement should contain vitamin C to aid absorption of the iron. Take a tissue salt called Ferrum Phos with your iron supplement. This will help your body absorb and utilise the iron in your supplement.

Cramps

During the third trimester your need for magnesium may increase by up to fifty per cent. Therefore, if cramps are becoming a problem, check your magnesium intake. Remember that you need at least 600 mg of magnesium each day. It is a difficult mineral to digest and is often lacking in our food supply. You might also need some extra calcium. If you are taking 600 mg of magnesium and 1200 mg of calcium daily and you still get cramps, you may not be digesting the minerals well. Take one tablet of Calc Phos and one tablet of Mag Phos four times a day. Cramps may suggest that all your minerals are low, so see your health practitioner.

Regular gentle exercise and massage can also help prevent cramps.

Cravings

Cravings often suggest a mineral deficiency. Take a multimineral supplement containing calcium, magnesium, manganese, molybdenum, zinc, copper, potassium and iron. If the cravings continue, see a naturopath.

Dental Problems and Sore Gums

Dental problems during pregnancy are a sign of inadequate nutrition or absorption of nutrients earlier in life. The growing baby will rapidly deplete a woman of nutrients if she has inadequate reserves. Minerals especially are lacking in our modern diets. Many people take extra vitamins, but they are unaware of the importance of minerals. Minerals, especially calcium and magnesium, are needed for bones and teeth, but are very difficult for us to digest, making it doubly difficult to obtain a sufficient supply. If you have a history of dental problems and frequent fillings, make sure you take a supplement giving you 1200 mg of calcium and 600 mg of magnesium daily.

Sore or bleeding gums often respond to extra vitamin C – 2000 to 3000 mg a day – and regular flossing. Take this high dose for a few days, then reduce it to 1000 mg each day and continue with this dosage. During pregnancy don't stop high doses of vitamin C quickly, always lower the dose over a period of a few days.

Make sure that you visit your dentist, but avoid unnecessary X-rays and fillings. Take the supplements recommended in the chapter on nutrition. Before any subsequent pregnancies, go on the complete pregnancy nutrition program for at least six months. This will build up your reserves of nutrients so that you are not drained by the next pregnancy.

Faintness

Faintness can be caused by low blood pressure which may occur early in pregnancy. It used to be the discreet Victorian woman's way of announcing to her husband that she was pregnant. If you do faint, make sure that you then stand up in stages slowly. Take 250 iu of vitamin E a day to help balance low blood pressure.

Fatigue

Tiredness is inevitable if you don't allow your body adequate rest time. You also need to eat good nourishing food and take supplements of B vitamins and iron if you are still struggling. Remember that some of your energy is being utilised for your growing child, so you may need more sleep than usual. Fatigue is more common in the early weeks and again in the later weeks of pregnancy.

Fluid Retention

This is common in late pregnancy. It affects especially the face, hands and ankles and is often aggravated in warm weather. Your doctor will check that you do not have pre-eclampsia. This is associated with high blood pressure, swollen ankles and the presence of protein in the urine. If pre-eclampsia is suspected or confirmed, you will need to be monitored carefully by your doctor.

If the swelling is not a sign of pre-eclampsia, there is much you can do to reduce the discomfort. Wear comfortable flat shoes. Rest with your feet up as often as you can. Regular walking helps keep fluid moving. Avoid tea, coffee, salty foods and foods high in sugar as these may increase fluid retention. Eat fresh celery regularly. Vitamin B6 reduces fluid retention, take 50 - 100 mg each day with your multi-B supplement. Dandelion leaf is a good diuretic and with its high potassium content does not cause a depletion of this mineral the way synthetic diuretics do. You may take it as capsules or as a tea.

Haemorrhoids

Constipation and relaxation of the intestinal muscles can contribute to the formation of haemorrhoids or piles. These are varicose veins in the anus, which can bleed, sometimes quite profusely. Do not allow yourself to become constipated. (See the section on constipation.) Eat plenty of high-fibre foods such as fresh fruit and vegetables, get some regular exercise such as walking, and drink at least eight glasses of water daily.

Haemorrhoids will often respond to witch-hazel, also known as hamamelis. You can buy this as an ointment to be applied topically, or you may need to visit a homoeopath if the problem does not resolve with these simple measures.

Headaches

The tissue salts Calc Phos and Mag Phos, one of each taken or chewed four times a day, can help with headaches. Both calcium and magnesium are required in large amounts during pregnancy and headaches will often respond to increased availability of these minerals.

A Bowen therapy treatment or osteopathic adjustment will often relieve pressure from a tight neck contributing to headaches.

If stress contributes to your headaches, you need to identify the source of the stress and take some stress relieving measures. Tai chi, yoga and massage may all help, as will adequate rest and a balanced lifestyle.

Sometimes headaches are the result of an allergy, often to dairy foods. In this case you need to see a practitioner.

Indigestion

Eat small meals often rather than a few large meals. This puts less pressure on your cramped digestive organs, and keeps your blood sugar more stable. Chamomile or peppermint tea sometimes helps. Make your own tea using the flowers as chamomile tea bags may not contain the active ingredients in sufficient quantities. Homoeopathic remedies such as Nux Vomica are safe and often very effective. See a practitioner if the problem persists.

Do not smoke as this affects digestion. Avoid spicy and fatty foods. Do not drink with meals as this may dilute your digestive juices and can leave some people feeling bloated.

Morning Sickness

The high levels of female hormones during pregnancy are believed to cause the nausea associated with the first trimester. Have a couple of dry biscuits or a small piece of fresh fruit on rising. It helps if these can be brought to you in bed. Avoid spicy and fatty foods. Eat small meals regularly during the day rather than two or three large ones.

Chamomile or peppermint tea can relieve the nausea. A few drops of peppermint oil on a cotton ball by the bed at night may help you wake feeling less nauseated.

If after these measures you still suffer morning sickness, take some ginger supplements for travel sickness available from a health food store. Ginger has been shown to be an effective and safe treatment for morning sickness. The tissue salt Kali Mur sometimes helps with morning sickness. If the nausea involves acid or sour reflux, try the tissue salt Nat Phos. If these measures fail, consider seeing a naturopath. Homoeopathic remedies such as Nux Vomica can help.

Vitamin B6 helps some women – take 25 mg every eight hours. I generally don't recommend taking B vitamins in isolation for any period of time. Take a multi-B vitamin that contains at least 50 mg of vitamin B6. You can then take extra vitamin B6 if necessary.

If the morning sickness is very severe, and you are considering future pregnancies, obtain some naturopathic advice before you become pregnant again.

Skin Problems

Skin problems may resolve or worsen during pregnancy. If you have a pre-existing skin problem, your need for good nutrition and extra supplementation is great indeed.

The essential fatty acids from linseed oil or a combination of evening primrose oil and the fish oils recommended in the chapter on nutrition generally help dry or oily skin problems. See a practitioner if skin problems persist.

Sleep Disturbances

Sleep is not always as restful as you need during pregnancy and perhaps this is nature's way of preparing you for disturbed nights once the baby is born. Whatever the reason, a few drops of essential oil of lavender in the bedroom at night can often help. Drink some chamomile tea early in the evening. The herbs hops, passionflower and valerian are also safe in pregnancy and lactation. They are recommended whenever there is restlessness, sleep disturbance and any nervous tension. These herbs are easily available from health food stores or you may wish to visit a practitioner. Take one tablet of passionflower or valerian about one hour before going to bed. This should have you sleeping well. The tissue salt Kali Phos is useful if you feel oversensitive and irritable with the sleeplessness.

Massage can help promote very deep and restful sleep. Encourage your partner to give you a back rub using a massage blend with essential oils (see chapter 4). Have a regular massage with a massage therapist. A warm bath or foot bath with a couple of added drops of lavender oil just before bedtime is also a wonderful way to encourage good sleep.

Don't drink liquids late at night and especially avoid tea and coffee in the evening. Coffee is stimulating, and both tea and coffee have diuretic effects. Disturbed sleep is often the result of the need to urinate during the night as the growing uterus crowds the bladder.

Stretch Marks

Stretch marks may appear wherever the skin needs to expand quickly. This may occur over your expanding tummy and breasts, but may also affect the thighs and upper arms. Daily massage with a moisturising blend will give the skin moisture to help it stretch. Massage with a good quality vitamin E cream or a blend of avocado or almond oil with essential oils of neroli, tangerine or lavender. While you are massaging your tummy each day, this is a great time to get in touch with your baby and enjoy this unique togetherness. Also consider massaging the perineum with the same vitamin E cream or with some jojoba oil. Studies have shown that regular perineal massage reduces the incidence of tearing and episiotomy.

If you have a regular massage during pregnancy, your therapist will also massage your tummy with a good moisturising blend.

Zinc and vitamins A and E during pregnancy give the skin the nutrition it needs. Amounts are recommended in the chapter on nutrition and supplements. Zinc especially is often lacking whenever skin does not stretch easily.

Thrush

Tendencies to thrush seem to be exaggerated during pregnancy because of the hormonal changes taking place. Thrush is caused by a yeast-like fungus called candida albicans. It thrives after antibiotic use, whenever the immune system is compromised, and when there are hormonal changes such as during pregnancy, menopause and the use of the contraceptive pill.

Take an acidophilus and bifidus supplement three times a day before meals. Yoghurt and yoghurt drinks are often not high enough in these beneficial bacteria to overcome a deep problem. Many yoghurt drinks are also high in sugar – candida's favourite food! Cut back on sugary and processed foods, and any yeast containing foods such as wine and mushrooms.

Avoid fruit and obtain your vitamins and carbohydrates from vegetables and grains. If you must have fruit, eat it after you have eaten other foods. This enables the fruit to be digested more slowly so that the fruit sugars are not released quickly into your system.

If thrush continues, see a practitioner, as the baby may be affected if thrush is present during the birth.

Varicose Veins

As with haemorrhoids, varicose veins are caused by relaxation in the vein walls during pregnancy. You have extra blood volume during pregnancy and the extra weight of pregnancy puts further strain on the blood supply to the legs. Regular gentle exercise, especially walking and swimming, helps keep the blood supply moving. Elevate your legs whenever you can, especially on hot days. Treatment is similar to that for haemorrhoids – witch-hazel as an ointment or taken homoeopathically.

Chapter 6

PREPARING FOR LABOUR

Pregnancy is sometimes referred to as a 'prelude to labour'. Throughout your pregnancy, your body sustains the growing foetus, but it also prepares for expulsion of the child at the end of the pregnancy. There are many things you can do to help the process of labour to be accomplished efficiently. These involve two main aspects. The first is knowledge and understanding of the process of labour. The second involves physical preparation beforehand to encourage, at full term, the most efficient labour possible for you. If after all this preparation, you still need pain killing medication or medical intervention, at least you will feel that you did the best you could, and that you have given your infant the best possible start in life. Unfortunately, some women need forceps, epidurals or a caesarean section even after adequate preparation, but you and your child will recover more quickly if you are in good health and have a full understanding of the procedure and its necessity.

Understanding the process of labour and what to expect empowers you. No two labours are the same, even for the same woman, except for the fact that a normally progressing labour has contractions steadily increasing in duration and intensity. Attend childbirth or prenatal classes to learn breathing techniques to use during the contractions. These classes are run by your hospital or birthing unit and give you vital information about labour and birth as well as providing contact with other pregnant women. Feeling in control of the situation and using the breathing techniques you have learnt will enable you to avoid or minimise the use of pain killing medications, which are known to affect the unborn child.

Strong and effective contractions shorten the length of time you need to be in labour. You will emerge from your labour without the exhaustion resulting from a long and stressful ordeal. Your preparation for labour will include adequate nutrition as discussed in the chapter on diet. Pregnancy is a time of heightened nutritional requirements both for yourself and for your child, so good nutrition before the birth will give you a sound basis for your own good health as well as the best health for your child.

Rest frequently in the days before your due date. Sleep is often not as refreshing as you might like, so you need to make up for it by some extra rest time. Also you may start labour during the night and the lost or disturbed sleep may make it more difficult for you to concentrate on your breathing techniques.

Gentle exercise such as walking, tai chi and some yoga exercises are all useful to keep you relaxed and calm during the last days of your pregnancy. Exercise helps keep you fit and contributes to good sleep. Continue whatever exercise program you have been following during your pregnancy, but you may need to take it much more slowly and gently as your pregnancy progresses.

To tone and strengthen the uterus there are some herbs you can use during the last months of the pregnancy. These have a long history of use in preparing the uterus for strong, coordinated contractions. Some of these herbs are also known to help prevent premature labour and to decrease the discomfort of Braxton Hicks contractions. You can also use essential oil blends and flower remedies to prepare for labour.

HERBS USED TO PREPARE FOR LABOUR

Red raspberry is the best known of the herbs used to prepare the uterus for labour. It strengthens and tones the uterus, so that contractions will be effective and efficient. It should be taken regularly during the third trimester for best effect. Red raspberry is readily available as a tea or in tablet form. Drink the tea or take one tablet two or three times every day for the best effect.

There are other herbs which are also recommended during the last three months of pregnancy. These herbs will tone the uterus for the work it will do during labour, but they also have properties which help the uterus to relax during pregnancy and have been used to decrease the risk of premature labour. In their capacity as relaxants, they can diminish the discomfort experienced during Braxton Hicks contractions. These are often painful and powerful contractions which occur during the last few weeks of pregnancy. The herbs recommended here include squaw vine, false unicorn root, black haw and cramp bark. You will need to obtain these herbs from a qualified naturopath or herbalist, who will also advise you on how to take them.

ESSENTIAL OILS

Use essential oils regularly during your pregnancy. Essential oils and massage are so beneficial and there is so much to say about them that they have been given a chapter of their own, so refer to chapter 4 for a complete description of essential oils and their uses. They relax and nurture you during your pregnancy. They can be used to help with a number of common complaints of pregnancy, such as backache and sleeplessness. The regular use of essential oils during pregnancy seems to help the mother develop an awareness of their healing properties so that they are much more effective during labour.

MASSAGE

Massage can be used during pregnancy to relax and nurture both you and your partner. Practising during pregnancy will also give your partner the confidence to use massage during labour to help keep you calm and relaxed between contractions.

Practise with your partner the following massage techniques. Using firm circular movements with the heel of the hand massage around the lower back. Concentrate on the buttocks and the sacrum, the large bone across the lower part of the back. Don't press on the spine as this can be painful. Gently massage the sides of the belly with the flat of your hand.

Foot massage is not for everyone, but for those who enjoy it it is wonderfully relaxing and refreshing. Use firm, even circular movements with the thumb or the heel of the hand on the padded parts of the toes and the feet. Be very gentle with the more tender arch area, as this may be very sensitive.

FLOWER REMEDIES

The best-known flower remedies are those discovered by the English physician, Dr Edward Bach. In the 1930s, he abandoned a lucrative medical practice to devote his life to finding plants with healing properties. Since that time, flower remedies have been discovered in other countries. Australia has its own Bush Flower Essences. Unlike herbal remedies, which we use mostly to affect the physical body, flower remedies bring healing to emotional states. They are very gentle, have no side effects, are very safe, but can be very powerful.

Dr Bach found 38 remedies, including some for fear, anxiety and worry. There are some that are particularly appropriate during pregnancy. These include Aspen, Clematis, Gentian, Heather, Hornbeam, Mimulus, Walnut and Wild Oat. The remedies suggested here have a great deal of use during pregnancy, but there are others. For a complete description of all the Bach flower remedies, see chapter 9.

Aspen is **for fear of the unknown.** It is used when we are afraid, but there is no known reason for the fear, perhaps just vague apprehension. It may be appropriate in a first pregnancy as the experience of labour and childbirth is as yet unknown. People are often very willing to share their unpleasant childbirth experiences, and these tales can lead to unnecessary fears in the first-time mother. If you know what you are afraid of, Mimulus is a better choice. If you are not sure whether to use Mimulus or Aspen, use Mimulus first for a couple of weeks. Then use Aspen for a couple of weeks. They are better not mixed together.

Clematis is used for that dreamy, unreal feeling that often accompanies pregnancy. **Daydreaming, absent-mindedness** and an inability to concentrate will often respond to Clematis.

Gentian can be used whenever there is a feeling of **discouragement and self-doubt,** perhaps about your ability to cope with the demands of new motherhood.

Heather can be used if you feel that you have **lost interest** in anything not associated with pregnancy. While pregnancy can be a time of introspection, and the feelings of self-interest are nature's way of ensuring that the pregnant woman looks after herself very well, this should not be at the expense of your previous hobbies and interests. You should not find yourself unable to become interested in other people and their lives, nor should you be constantly talking only about issues related to pregnancy and childbirth. Heather can bring back your sense of perspective.

Hornbeam will bring strength to the **weariness and fatigue** often associated with pregnancy, especially if you are also coping with other small children. If you desperately need to rest, you must find the time for this whenever you can, or get some help so you can rest and be left in peace. However, Hornbeam will help give you strength to keep going until you can take that much needed rest.

Mimulus is another remedy for **fear** but, in contrast to Aspen, this time you know what the fear is about. It may be fear of your changing emotions or fear of a caesarean section. Mimulus may be useful in a subsequent pregnancy where an earlier labour has left unpleasant memories. If Mimulus does not help after a couple of weeks, try taking Aspen for a couple of weeks. Sometimes our fears are not what we think they are!

Walnut is needed in any **time of change** and this is certainly a big change in your life! It helps you establish new patterns of behaviour appropriate to your new circumstances. This remedy will also be useful for the newborn baby as well as during teething, adolescence, any career change or move to a new home.

Wild Oat may be helpful if you are not completely sure that you have made the right decision in becoming pregnant. Perhaps you are still unsure that you wish to give up your career and pursue motherhood. Wild Oat helps with **unresolved decisions,** whatever they are related to.

Other flower remedies may be useful depending on your own circumstances and your reaction to the ones I have mentioned. You might like to see a naturopath to help you choose flower remedies to suit you. There are also several books about Bach flowers if you wish to explore further the use of flower remedies.

If you do not achieve the desired effect with your chosen flower remedy, there may be others more appropriate for you. It may be necessary for you to see a practitioner. If the problem is a serious one, do not try to solve it on your own. Do not use flower remedies in place of appropriate professional help. Make sure you see a counsellor.

Rescue Remedy

Rescue Remedy is a combination of five of the Bach flower remedies. These are Cherry Plum for desperation, Clematis for inattentiveness and lack of concentration, Impatiens for impatience, Rock Rose for terror and Star of Bethlehem for shock. As the name suggests, Rescue Remedy is used whenever there is a crisis, upset or upheaval of any sort. Useful at any time, think of Rescue Remedy after bad news, whenever there is fright or fear, or if you are struggling to cope for any reason. It is also recommended during and after childbirth.

Rescue Remedy is a good, all-purpose remedy to have around. It is a useful one to use if you are unsure which flower remedies would help. You could start your flower remedy collection with Rescue Remedy. It is easily available and covers many circumstances. The Australian bush flower equivalent is Emergency Essence, if you prefer to use native Australian remedies.

Using Bach Flower Remedies

To use flower remedies you need just a couple of drops of the remedy. Use one remedy on its own or mix together up to four. Do not use more than four at a time as they generally seem to work better if just a few are chosen carefully. (Rescue Remedy is an exception to this.) You can take the remedy either straight from the dosage bottle or you can add a drop to a drink of water or juice and sip on the drink slowly. Generally, they need to be used four times a day for best effect, but can be used more often if necessary. Rescue Remedy can be used every ten or fifteen minutes if needed. Sometimes you will notice the effect immediately, but it may take some time if the problem is deeply entrenched.

TALKING, MUSIC AND OTHER SOUNDS

During your pregnancy, talk and sing to your baby, especially during quiet times and when you are relaxing. Encourage your partner and other children to do the same. Babies will recognise and respond to voices, music and sounds they have heard while still in the womb. Studies have shown that babies exposed to music before birth learn to recognise their favourite pieces and will show a preference for them after birth.

Music can be a highly emotional and moving experience. Remember your response to a stirring national anthem or to any well-known and well-loved piece of music. Music has been shown to increase the growth of plants, to aid concentration, to encourage sleep, and to help the recall of memorable or not-so-memorable circumstances. The aim during pregnancy is to use music to evoke calming, gentle and loving thoughts for both yourself and your new child.

Playing soft, gentle music during pregnancy is beneficial both to you and to your unborn child. Use music during relaxation, during massage, and when practising your breathing techniques for labour. While your choice of music is largely a personal selection, quiet, rather than loud music, is usually preferable. You need music which does not demand your attention in any way.

If you don't already have some personal favourites, experiment with slow classical music, especially music from the Baroque period. Known as the original 'mood music', this music stirs the emotions. The most famous composers include Bach, Beethoven, Handel, Haydn and Mozart, but there are others. If this field is new to you, listen to some classical music stations and write down the names of selections which appeal to you. You will be surprised at how quickly you begin to recognise your own preferences.

New Age music is readily available and is also very soothing and not demanding in any way, or you may have your own favourites. Remember that this is your personal choice, select whatever is soothing and pleasant for you.

If possible, you might also play this music during your labour. Some birthing units will allow you to choose your own music. This is something you will need to determine when you book in. If the music is familiar to you and has been playing while you have been relaxing during your pregnancy, it will remind you of these relaxed states and aid your relaxation during labour. Your baby will also be welcomed with music familiar from the time in the womb. Babies are soothed by music and voices which they have experienced before birth.

OTHER TREATMENTS

Bowen therapy, massage, acupuncture or Reiki treatments during your pregnancy prepare you for labour in a number of ways. They nurture you, keep you relaxed and aid sleep. They ensure that you are fit and well, and used to relaxing when you go into labour. They can prevent or minimise a number of aches and pains that might otherwise bother you in pregnancy. Bowen therapy and Reiki can help with emotional blocks which might be preventing you from enjoying your pregnancy fully, and help release fears associated with labour.

BIRTH KITS

During late pregnancy prepare your personal birth kit. Visit a herbalist, homoeopath or naturopath a month or two before your due date to seek advice on preparations appropriate to your needs. You will be advised on and provided with homoeopathic remedies, Bach flower remedies and/or herbal preparations for use during labour.

OVERDUE

If your due date comes and goes with no sign of any 'action', several possibilities will be suggested to you. Always be guided by your doctor about when to consider induction. Generally an induced birth is less comfortable, the contractions are stronger and you need to wear a drip, which limits your movement. The insertion of a drip also has the effect of making you feel that something is wrong, as we associate medical intervention with illness. Labour is not an illness, just a healthy body doing something very normal.

There are some things you could try before considering induction. Adequate nutrition before and during pregnancy and regular use of the appropriate herbs in the last trimester are the best preparation for a normal length pregnancy and for integrity of the placenta.

Wait at least one to two weeks before becoming concerned, as long as your doctor is happy that the placenta is still functioning well. Some babies just need a little longer than others. Check your due date carefully before you attempt to hurry things along.

If everything is fine and you wish to help things along, there are some simple measures you can take. Breast stimulation has been demonstrated to induce uterine contractions in some women. Stimulate the breasts regularly during the day as often as you think about it. Intercourse and orgasm will sometimes stimulate a uterus ready to start contractions. Try a relaxing massage, a Bowen therapy treatment or acupuncture. The homoeopathic remedy Caulophyllum can be taken regularly and sometimes helps. A herbalist or naturopath might give you herbs known to stimulate labour and some flower remedies which can remove emotional blocks to starting labour. These will be chosen specifically for you and your circumstances. A therapist will also talk to you about any fears or apprehensions you may have. Sometimes these are well hidden and while you may feel excited about the impending birth, you may also harbour fears and uncertainties.

Chapter 7

LABOUR AND BIRTH

Finally the long awaited day has arrived. Time to put everything you have learnt into practice. You will be able to use your well-rehearsed breathing techniques, your essential oils, flower remedies, your prepared herbs or homoeopathic support remedies. Your partner will know how to massage your back, and how to use any drops or essential oils you have chosen. Many of these supporting remedies and techniques are discussed in this chapter to help you decide which are appropriate for you and your circumstances.

Make sure that you have everything prepared ahead of time, packed and labelled. When booking your hospital stay, you will have checked whether you will be able to supply your own music, your choice of essential oils, and whether you will be able to use your herbal or homoeopathic support remedies. Ensure that you are quite clear about the use of baths, so that you avoid disappointment or confusion at a time when you need to feel calm and focussed.

If you have followed the good health guidelines, you will be rested and in good health when your labour starts. During labour move around as much as possible, especially during early labour. Movement has been shown to decrease the length of labour as gravity puts foetal pressure on the cervix and increases the size of the pelvic outlet.

ESSENTIAL OILS IN LABOUR

Essential oils have been found to have great benefits for the mother in labour. These benefits are greater if the mother has used oils throughout her pregnancy. Previous experience with them seems to familiarise the body with their calming and strengthening properties. During the last weeks of pregnancy you will have been massaging your tummy with oil blends, your partner will have been massaging you, and you will have experienced the oils around your home. It is very welcoming for a baby to be greeted by comforting aromas, especially if some of these have been experienced while in the womb. As well as their comforting and nurturing qualities, oils also offer antiseptic properties.

Always make sure that essential oils are mixed thoroughly in the bath or massage blend before use. In the labour room, use only a few drops of your oils as too much can leave your attendants feeling spaced out.

Have your blend prepared and labelled before you go into labour. Make sure that the instructions for use are clearly shown on the bottle and that your partner knows what to do. You may buy a ready-made blend or prepare your own with your favourite oils.

Essential oils have been discussed fully in chapter 4, but some are included here specifically for their use in labour:

- *Clary Sage.* Clary sage is a uterine tonic with uplifting effects. It is an antidepressant oil. It encourages labour while helping the mother to relax. Clary sage helps breathing and helps calm the mind, especially if there is any sense of panic. Use only small amounts of clary sage, as it can make everyone feel a little headachy, drowsy or 'off the planet'. Use in massage blends and compresses for the back and tummy.
- *Geranium.* An antidepressant oil with calming and uplifting effects, it is useful in anxiety states. It stimulates the circulation, so use in massage and lower back compresses. An excellent oil to use after the birth to stimulate the uterus to return to its normal size.
- *Lavender.* A calming and widely used oil, lavender is readily available, relatively inexpensive and generally popular. It is also a good antiseptic, has normalising properties and helps to increase the effect but not the pain of contractions.
- *Neroli.* Neroli has a very calming and soothing effect. It

helps allay fear and allows you to concentrate on the task at hand. Especially useful during the transition stage to calm and help avoid hyperventilation. It is a very expensive oil, but is available in some blends.

- *Rose.* Rose is especially useful during and after labour, with its strong affinity for the reproductive system and its toning and cleansing effect on the uterus. Calming and soothing, it encourages deep breathing and has strong antidepressant properties. Use in the bath or in massage blends.
- *Ylang Ylang.* Another calming oil which is useful to have in the labour room with its soothing and relaxing properties. Use in the bath or on a compress.

Bath

Early in labour have a bath with a few added drops of lavender oil. (If you intend to deliver in the bath, do not add essential oils as there is a risk that they might not be completely dispersed in the bath water and some undiluted oil may enter the baby's eyes.) Some hospitals and birthing units allow you to stay in the bath right up to and during delivery, others don't. Make sure you are informed about your choices when you book. Labour is not the time to find that you cannot do what you had planned nor the time to have an argument about it.

Compresses

Soak a small towel or face washer in warm water to which have been added a couple of drops of lavender, clary sage or rose. This can be held against your abdomen or your lower back if needed. If you are feeling hot, a cool compress with a drop of lavender or neroli is very refreshing.

After the Birth

After the birth, a drop of neroli or lavender under your pillow will help you relax, especially if you are exhausted but too overwhelmed or excited to sleep.

HOMOEOPATHIC REMEDIES

Homoeopathic remedies are specially prepared to be safe, gentle and effective. They are prepared with very small quantities of the substance to be used, which makes them very safe for use in pregnancy, labour and even with very young babies. There are several to choose from that are appropriate for labour. You will need to obtain these from a qualified homoeopath or purchase a pre-prepared homoeopathic birth kit.

Homoeopathic remedies are very sensitive to heat and light and must be stored carefully. They must also be kept away from strong smells such as essential oils. This means that if you are using both, wash your hands well after handling oils and before using homoeopathic remedies, and store them separately.

- *Caulophyllum* is the best known of all the homoeopathic remedies for childbirth. It ensures effective and regular contractions and can be used if contractions diminish in regularity and strength. It is also recommended that you take a few drops of Caulophyllum each day during the last couple of weeks of pregnancy, especially if you have not been using the preparatory herbs such as red raspberry.
- *Arnica* is especially useful for both mother and baby after the birth as it helps the healing of any bruising and trauma. Bruising may not always be obvious, but the process of labour and delivery is highly likely to lead to bruised tissue in mother and child, especially if the birth was quick, if forceps were used or if tissue was torn. Arnica is easily available and is a good remedy to have at home in your First Aid kit. You will need to see a homoeopath for other homoeopathic remedies appropriate for labour and birth.

Use only a few drops of a homoeopathic remedy under the tongue or in a small glass of water. As these remedies must be kept away from strong odours, have them about fifteen minutes before you eat or drink, brush your teeth or chew gum. Store them separately from your essential oils.

FLOWER REMEDIES

There are flower remedies for a number of emotional states and you may have been using them already during your pregnancy. If you have already used them, you will enter labour much calmer and more relaxed than you might have been otherwise. If some of the flower remedies worked especially well for you during your pregnancy, they may also be very helpful during labour. Rescue Remedy is especially useful for mother, father and baby during and after the birth. Aspen, Gentian, Hornbeam and Walnut have been discussed in chapter 6.

You need just a drop of the flower remedy. You can take it either straight from the dosage bottle or you can add a drop to a drink of water and sip slowly. It can also be placed on a pulse point, for example, at the wrist.

Other flower remedies which may be useful during labour include:

- *Rock Rose.* This remedy is for very great fear and terror, for nightmares. It may be useful towards the end of the first stage of labour, when your emotions can become quite strong and overwhelming. Rock Rose is included in Rescue Remedy.
- *Impatiens.* As its name suggests, Impatiens is for people who become tense and anxious and perhaps even angry if they have to wait. This could be a useful remedy during the last days of pregnancy and during early labour if things are taking a little while to get going. Impatiens is included in Rescue Remedy.
- *Elm.* Elm gives strength at times when we may temporarily feel overwhelmed and unable to continue. If you feel that you are unable to go on because the task is just too daunt-

ing, Elm can restore your sense of purpose and self-confidence. This could be useful at any time during labour, but especially if you feel that you have been there forever and still have a few centimetres to dilate. It also helps to remember that the speed of dilation increases as you go further into labour. Therefore, the last few centimetres generally take a lot less time than the first few.

- *Star of Bethlehem.* This is specifically for shock and its numbing effects. Give to the baby after birth. Also useful for the mother if she is stunned or exhausted after the birth. Star of Bethlehem is included in Rescue Remedy.

Babies and children respond very well to flower remedies and I suggest that they have some specially chosen for them soon after birth.

HERBS

There are several herbs which can help make labour efficient (see chapter 3). You will need to visit a naturopath or herbalist for these. Herbs used might include blue cohosh, black cohosh, cramp bark, raspberry leaves, motherwort, wild yam or chamomile. If you have a history of difficult breastfeeding, include separately some blessed thistle, chaste tree and raspberry leaves for use after the birth.

CHECKLIST

As well as the paraphernalia your hospital or birthing unit has recommended, check that you have included any of the following that you have chosen to use during your labour:

- Essential oils.
- Homoeopathic or herbal preparations to encourage labour and aid relaxation between contractions.
- Rescue Remedy or other Bach flower remedies.

- Music.
- Raspberry leaves as a tea or tablet to stimulate milk supply and tone the uterus and pelvic muscles after the birth.

Ensure that everything is labelled with your name and instructions for use, although, ideally, by now your partner will know what oils and remedies you have chosen and how to use them. He or she will then be able to take charge of them for you. Include your contact telephone number to ensure that everything is returned to you in case you forget something at the hospital or birthing centre.

Chapter 8

HOME WITH THE BABY

Caring for your new baby also involves caring for yourself. Maintain your good health with plenty of fresh foods, plenty of rest and the healthy attitude that you carried throughout your pregnancy.

Continue on the healthy diet you have followed during your pregnancy. Avoid alcohol, processed foods and foods that are high in sugar or fat. Also continue with the supplements you were taking before the birth. Your baby will still take all his nutrition from you through your breast milk. Breastfeeding women often find that they also need to avoid spicy foods; too much fruit; and foods that cause wind such as cabbage, lentils or onions. Coffee, chocolate, eggs and tomatoes may also cause problems such as colic.

Breastfeed for as long as you are able. Breastfeeding has been shown to decrease the incidence of asthma and other allergies and to protect the baby's delicate immune system against pathogens. Breast milk is much easier for your baby to digest and assimilate than formula milk, and is convenient and hygienic.

If you choose not to breastfeed, or find that you cannot, you can still care for and nurture yourself and your family. Continue to eat well to ensure that you are healthy and able to meet the demands of motherhood.

Although it may often be difficult to find the time when you are home with a new baby, it is important that you still nurture yourself. Rest whenever you have the opportunity. Continue with your massage, regular gentle exercise, listening to favourite music, or any other simple ways you have found to take care of yourself. Go for easy and gentle walks. Practise your pelvic floor exercises (see the following section) regularly to tone more quickly the muscles stretched by childbirth. It is too easy to fall into the trap of rushing around all the time looking after others and forgetting to take care of your own needs. Ignoring your need for rest and relaxation will lead to emotional and physical exhaustion.

PELVIC FLOOR (KEGEL) EXERCISES

The pelvic floor is made up of bands of muscles which support the structures in the pelvis. Strong pelvic floor muscles maintain the bladder, uterus and bowel in their correct positions and enable them to function properly. Weakened pelvic floor muscles may contribute to stress incontinence. This causes uncontrollable leakage or loss of urine on coughing, laughing, walking or running, jumping, sneezing or lifting. If you have to wear a pad because of uncontrollable urine leakage or have to cross your legs to prevent urine flow when laughing, coughing or sneezing, you may have stress incontinence. Almost half of all pregnant women may experience some degree of stress incontinence because increased pressure on the pelvic floor stretches the muscles. Constipation, common in pregnancy, may also contribute to decreased pelvic muscle tone. Childbirth may further weaken the ligaments and muscles which maintain the bladder in its correct position.

Other symptoms which may suggest weakened pelvic floor muscles include: urgency of bladder emptying or bowel movements, decreased sensation in the vagina or a feeling of something in the vagina. Prolapse may occur several years after child bearing if there is serious or prolonged relaxation of the pelvic floor muscles. A prolapse involves the bulging of the bladder, uterus or bowel into the vagina as a result of poor muscle tone and the resulting relaxation of the organs.

To strengthen the pelvic floor, thereby strengthening the muscles which support the bladder, uterus and bowel, Kegel or pelvic floor exercises were developed. Regular practice of these exercises reduces the incidence of stress incontinence, protects against prolapse and improves the tone of the vagina, increasing sexual sensation. To identify the appropriate muscles you need to be familiar with three groups of muscles. To find the first muscle group, stop your urine flow in midstream. The second group tightens around your vagina. You should be able to feel a squeezing movement when you insert two fingers. The third muscle group can be found by tightening your anus as if you are trying to stop wind passing. These groups of muscles are the ones which support the pelvic floor. Now that you are able to identify these muscles, practise contracting them all at the same time. Bring the muscles upwards slowly and hold at maximum contraction for a count of five to ten, then slowly relax them. It may help to imagine these muscles as an elevator or a lift travelling upwards. Bring the lift up from the ground floor to the first, second, third and finally fourth floors. Repeat this ten times. Practise regularly several times a day. You will find it easier to remember to do the Kegel exercises if you have a regular routine for doing them. Practise them when stopped at a traffic light, when at the kitchen sink, after urinating or when watching commercials on television. The exercises become easier the more often you practise. It may take a little while, up to a few weeks or even several months, to notice an improvement if the muscles are very weakened. Persist, as the results will be worth the effort.

While doing the exercises, do not hold your breath or tense your stomach muscles. If you are doing them correctly, you also won't feel any tightening of your thighs or buttock muscles. Occasionally practise the exercises standing up as this is when the stress on the pelvic floor muscles is greatest. Do not restrict fluids in an effort to minimise stress incontinence. This will only make you more susceptible to other bladder problems, including infection. It is best not to practise these exercises while you are urinating, but after you have finished is a good time as you can make this a regular routine.

If you have difficulties with the exercises or you do not notice any improvement in your symptoms after two or three months of regular practice, consult a physiotherapist or your doctor.

ESSENTIAL OILS

Keep using your essential oils around the house in a burner, vaporiser or in a saucer with warm water. Use them to keep the house smelling fragrant, to keep germs at bay, to lift your moods, to encourage restful sleep and for anything else you like.

I don't recommend using essential oils in a young baby's bath as there is a risk that some undiluted oil will get in the eyes or that the oil will not disperse properly through the bath. Oils can be used safely in a massage blend if mixed thoroughly, but avoid oil on the baby's hands in case they end up in his mouth. Thoroughly mix one drop only of the chosen oil in about 20 ml of almond or jojoba oil. Do not use baby oil as it leaches vitamins from the skin. To make a cream, choose a bland unscented cream base which doesn't contain lanolin. Allow one drop of essential oil to 20 ml of cream and mix thoroughly.

Essential oils recommended for babies include any of the oils recommended during pregnancy and labour. Pure essential oils of chamomile or neroli are preferable to the two per cent blends with jojoba. These blends may be cheaper, but they do not have the strength of the therapeutic properties of pure chamomile or neroli oil. You may also use clary sage, geranium, lavender, neroli, rose or sandalwood.

HERBS

For yourself, continue using the herbs you used during your pregnancy. These will help balance your hormones, ensuring that fluctuating hormones do not cause you continuing problems. For example, raspberry helps tone the uterus and enhances your milk supply.

Herbs which can be used safely for babies include chamomile flowers, peppermint leaves and melissa. For a herbal preparation of chamomile, choose chamomile extract or loose chamomile flowers, not tea bags. The tea bags may not contain the active ingredients in sufficient quantities. Allow one tablespoon of the extract for each two litres of water for a bath or rinse. If you are using the flowers, make a strong tea using two tablespoons, then add to the baby's bath.

SOME COMMON PROBLEMS

Breastfeeding

The advantages of breastfeeding have been promoted frequently. Breast milk is the ideal food, it is fast, sterile, there is no preparation involved and it offers perfect nutrition for the baby. It contains important antibodies to protect and support the baby's immature immune system and reduces the incidence of allergies. Breastfeeding promotes mother-baby interaction. For the mother, it helps the uterus to regain its pre-pregnant tone. Oxytocin, one of the hormones involved in milk production, is also called the 'feel good' hormone and is known for its role in reducing anxiety and promoting a feeling of well-being.

Prolactin and oxytocin are the two main hormones involved in the production of breast milk. Prolactin production increases with the decline in levels of oestrogen and progesterone after the birth. This hormone produces milk and is stimulated by suckling. Levels fluctuate during the day and are highest at night. The other hormone, oxytocin, produces the let-down reflex caused by the contraction of tiny muscles around the milk glands. This has the effect of releasing most of the milk. Levels of oxytocin are also stimulated by the baby's feeding and any nipple stimulation, and they rise and fall in waves during the day. Supply of breast milk is very much a function of demand. Regular and frequent nursing will stimulate levels of both hormones necessary for milk production. To establish and maintain an adequate milk supply it is necessary to nurse regularly. Avoid stress, get plenty of rest and maintain a nutritious and satisfying diet. Hormone levels may drop if you do not nurse frequently. You may also reduce your milk supply if you attempt to diet or restrict your fluid intake, if you are very tired and stressed, if you become anxious about breastfeeding or if you conceive again.

Your midwife will help you with breastfeeding posture and technique. Once you are home, there are many organisations which promote and encourage breastfeeding. Contact one near you for valuable help, advice and support. These organisations are also a useful way of meeting other new mothers.

Use the time while feeding your baby as a time together, to talk and cuddle. It is a time to provide both physical and emotional nourishment to your child. It is a very precious time for bonding and for interaction between mother and baby. This is true irrespective of whether you breast or bottle-feed or use a combination of both. If you have some concerns about your breastfeeding, try concentrating on the positive emotional aspects of feeding. This will relax you, enable you to enjoy the experience and will encourage greater success than if you focus only on the mechanics of feeding.

Breast Engorgement

Two to five days after the birth, milk production and increased blood supply to the breasts can cause painful swelling or engorgement. It generally settles down after a few days, but it can be very uncomfortable and may continue past the first few days. Warm or cold compresses of geranium, rose or lavender essential oils can be used regularly. The tissue salt Kali Mur is useful for swelling. Putting fresh cabbage leaves inside the bra is an old but not very effective remedy.

If the nipples crack, if you are prone to mastitis or if your breasts start to feel hot, drink dandelion root tea regularly during the day. It is used in China for mastitis. Also take echinacea, garlic and extra vitamin C to prevent an infection setting in. Use the same tissue salts you would use for any inflammation. Use Ferrum Phos in the early stages and Kali Mur for swelling. Cracked nipples need Ferrum Phos, Calc Fluor and Silica. Take your chosen tissue salts every hour during the early stages of inflammation, then four times a day until the symptoms have gone completely.

Colds and Flu

If anyone in the household comes home with a cold or the flu, or if flu is rampant while your baby is young and has an immature immune system, there are a number of things you can do to minimise the risk of your baby or yourself contracting the virus. Use essential oils of eucalyptus, pine or peppermint in a burner or vaporiser or use a drop on a cotton ball placed in the living room and bedrooms. These oils help with breathing and have been shown to be useful in ensuring that the infections are not transferred to other family members.

Take some echinacea yourself to minimise your risk of infection and to boost your own immune system. Alternatively, take 2000 mg of vitamin C each day.

The tissue salts Kali Mur and Ferrum Phos can be taken to reduce symptoms if you do succumb to a cold. Take them hourly at first, then four times a day until you feel completely well.

Homoeopathic remedies are safe and effective during lactation and for babies. Some are available over the counter, but you may choose to visit a homoeopath or naturopath.

Colic

Colic is caused by painful spasms of the digestive tract. If your baby is at all colicky, eat a diet based on fresh foods with adequate amounts of protein, lots of vegetables and grains such as rice, oats and barley. Consume as little processed food as possible and avoid coffee. Minimise wheat and dairy foods, as these are often the culprits in various allergies. Have a lactation consultant check your technique because colic may be a reaction to feeding too quickly. Also make sure that you give the baby plenty of time to burp to remove any wind accumulated during the feed.

Chamomile flowers, fennel and peppermint are the recommended first line treatments for colic. Make sure that you use chamomile flowers, not chamomile tea bags as these usually do not contain sufficient amounts of the active ingredients. Drink teas made of these and use the essential oils in a massage blend for the baby. If either of you is tense about feeding, add some hops to your tea blend.

Colic will sometimes respond to bifidobacterium infantis given to the baby before a feed. This is similar to acidophilus and bifidus, but bifidobacterium infantis is more prevalent in a baby's digestive system.

Tummy massage has been shown in a Danish study to reduce colic symptoms. Use a massage blend with essential oil of peppermint, fennel or chamomile. Hold the baby face downwards in your lap. Using a broad stroke with the flat of your hand, move in ever increasing circles around the abdomen. Make your strokes up on the baby's right and down on the left to take advantage of the direction of the large intestine. This is recommended about fifteen minutes after a feed. If you feel you need some help with your technique, visit a professional massage therapist. There are also courses available in baby massage.

Gentle cranial osteopathy helps sometimes. You might also wish to use some of the homoeopathic colic and indigestion blends available.

If colic continues despite these measures or beyond the third month, you will need to have the baby assessed for more serious conditions, such as allergy or digestive problems.

Cracked Nipples

Ensure that you have the correct feeding technique and that the baby is positioned and feeding properly. Apply honey to the nipples between feeds. This will soothe the area and honey has some antiseptic properties. Another preparation which sometimes helps is aloe vera gel to which you have added one drop of rose essential oil or calendula. Apply to the nipple and areola after each feed. Make sure that you wash off any preparation thoroughly before your baby feeds. Allow the nipples to air frequently and do not use soap on them as this can be very drying.

Use the tissue salts Ferrum Phos, Calc Fluor and Silica. These need to be taken every hour initially, then four times a day until the nipples have healed completely.

Take echinacea, garlic and extra vitamin C to prevent an infection setting in.

Cradle Cap

Cradle cap is the itching, scaling crusts which sometimes form on the baby's scalp. Chamomile oil in a base of jojoba oil can be massaged into the area regularly. Witch-hazel (also known as hamamelis) ointment has also been used successfully. Creams of viola tricolor or wild pansy can be used. Increase your own intake of the essential fatty acids in linseed oil or a combination of evening primrose oil and fish oil.

Dry Skin

An infusion of chamomile flowers in the bath is a recommended method for moisturising a baby's dry and sensitive skin. Chamomile massage blends and ointments are more concentrated, but they too can be used. Calendula and witch-hazel (or hamamelis) ointments are also safe and easily available.

Episiotomy

If you have had a tear or an episiotomy, wash the area with warm water to which you have added a drop of lavender oil. This will stimulate healing of the perineum and reduce the risk of infection. The same rinse can be used after a caesarean section to help the wound heal. Also continue to take your homoeopathic Arnica regularly to help with any bruising you have experienced. Zinc and vitamins A and C help with wound healing. Take 10 - 15 mg of zinc, 2000 mg of vitamin C and 5000 iu of vitamin A each day.

Insufficient Milk

Make sure you eat well and rest often. You need plenty of calories to maintain a good milk supply and to maintain your own nourishment. Now is not the time to start dieting. If you are at all stressed, your milk will dry up quickly. Well-meaning friends and relatives can make you feel totally inadequate and encourage switching to a bottle formula. Trust your own instincts. If you wish to persevere with breastfeeding, get some advice from a lactation consultant. She will check that your positioning is correct, that you are relaxed and eating well. She will also be a good source of sensible advice and reassurance.

Avoid tea and coffee as both are diuretics. Caffeine also decreases prolactin levels. Feed your baby regularly as this stimulates milk production. Drink plenty of filtered water. Herbs such as blessed thistle, raspberry leaves, vitex agnus castus and goat's rue can be used to boost your milk supply. Raspberry leaf tea was recommended before birth, so continue with your routine. Drink at least three cups each day or continue with the tablets. Blessed thistle and vitex agnus castus are easily available.

Essential oils of geranium or clary sage in a massage blend can also help. Make sure that these are washed off thoroughly before each feed. An old remedy, which supposedly draws fluids towards the breast, involves rubbing a few drops of castor oil into the area around the nipple after each feed.

Mastitis

Bacteria entering through cracked nipples or from inflammation from a blocked milk duct may cause infection in the breast. Cracked nipples should be prevented using the measures described under the heading 'Cracked Nipples'. To avoid blocked milk ducts, feed the baby regularly and follow the suggestions under the heading 'Breast Engorgement'. Mastitis often presents with fever, breast tenderness and redness. Dandelion root tea is used in China for mastitis. Drink a cup regularly during the day. Do not use the dandelion coffee preparations. These have low levels of the active ingredients. Obtain the root to prepare your tea or obtain a herbal extract. Mastitis can also be treated as you would treat any other infection. The herb echinacea is useful; in this case use the strongest preparation available. Take extra vitamin C and garlic. The tissue salts Kali Mur and Ferrum Phos used regularly every hour during the early stages may help the body deal with infection. Silica helps the cracked nipples to heal. Wash and air dry the nipples and apply aloe vera gel or witch-hazel ointment.

Nappy Rash

Nappy rash is often caused by a type of dermatitis. Prevention by regular nappy changing, keeping the baby's bottom clean and dry, and the use of soothing ointments is much better than treating a severe case of nappy rash. Allow the baby's skin time to be in contact with fresh air in a warm room. Don't use talcum powder as this cakes on the skin and can contribute to the problem by holding moisture next to the skin. Ensure that cloth nappies are rinsed properly after washing to avoid soap build-up.

Chamomile flowers can be used as an infusion and as an ointment. Use chamomile flowers to make an infusion for the bath and the extract of chamomile to make a rinse to be used after nappy changing. Use pawpaw ointment after you have washed and dried the area well. If you wish to use essential oils, add a drop of chamomile essential oil to a base oil such as jojoba or almond, or mix into a bland moisturising cream. Zinc creams, too, are a good base; use the white ones, not the coloured ones used as sunscreens. If you are breastfeeding, increase your intake of linseed oil or take essential fatty acids in the form of evening primrose oil and fish oil. Take two table-spoons of linseed oil or 2000 mg each of fish oil and evening primrose oil.

Nappy rash caused by allergy or an immature digestive system will sometimes respond to bifidobacterium infantis given to the baby before a feed, especially if there is some colic as well.

If the rash continues in spite of your best efforts, you may need to check whether allergies are the cause.

Postnatal Depression

Hopefully, if you have followed the advice given about good care during your pregnancy, you will not experience this upsetting and draining condition. If, despite your best efforts, you still have trouble getting out of the baby blues, continue your super nutritious diet and supplements. Take female herbs such as vitex agnus castus. Use neroli and petitgrain essential oils in a bath, shower or massage blend. Make sure that you get plenty of rest and get some fresh air and exercise every day. Take your baby for a walk. Exercise releases hormones that contribute to feelings of wellbeing. Get a massage from a pro-fessional therapist. Do not be afraid to ask for help with daily household chores or with other small children.

St John's wort, otherwise known as hypericum, has received a lot of attention lately as a safe and reliable alterna-tive to prescription antidepressants. It can aid sleep, relieve depression and promote a feeling of wellbeing. Unlike pre-scription drugs, it does not leave you feeling spaced out and it does not interfere with your sleep patterns. Take 2000 mg a day to start with. This can be increased if you feel this dose is not enough, but get some professional advice from a naturopath or herbalist before you do. Decrease to 1000 mg each day once you have started to feel better.

Rescue Remedy and other Bach flower remedies can be useful. Take the Rescue Remedy frequently straight from the bottle or in a drink.

There are also homoeopathic remedies which can help with stress and depression. You may need to see a qualified naturopath or homoeopath for these.

If your depression continues, seek professional help.

Sleeplessness

On average, newborn babies sleep for a total of about seventeen hours each day. Young babies alternate between periods of wakefulness and periods of sleep during the day and night. As they grow their sleep patterns change and by the age of about six months there should be a long stretch of sleep at night with two shorter sleeps during the day. At this age they need about fourteen hours of sleep each day. Babies are considered to be sleeping through the night if they have five hours of uninterrupted sleep.

Babies spend about half of their sleep time in an active sleep state. This stage of sleep is thought to be necessary for growth and development. The active state is a stage of sleep where there is fine muscular twitching and irregular breathing and the baby may cry out but remain asleep. There are rapid eye movements and dreaming is thought to occur during this stage of sleep. There may be easy waking during this active stage. The rest of the sleep time is spent in deep or quiet sleep, with some transitional time between the two stages. Deep sleep is characterised by regular breathing and no eye movements. During this stage of sleep it will be much more difficult to wake the baby.

From birth to six months of age babies will generally wake two or three times during the night. This frequency decreases to once or twice during the night until one year of age, and perhaps once during the night until two years of age. Evening is the most restless time for many babies, with more fussiness and crying than during other times of the day. Very young babies will wake regularly to feed. Breastfed babies may want to feed every couple of hours. Bottle-fed babies may need to be fed less often.

These are average times and any individual baby will have his own unique habits. Just as adults differ in their sleep patterns, so do babies differ in both the amount of time they spend in sleep and in their patterns of sleep. Some establish regular sleeping habits by the time they are only a few weeks old whereas others take much longer and may cause many frustrations and sleepless nights for their parents. Be prepared for your baby to wake regularly and do not assume adult patterns of sleep soon after birth. If your baby is waking regularly during the night, this does not necessarily represent an abnormal pattern. Keep a record of your baby's sleep habits; you may be surprised to find that the pattern is a normal one for the baby's age. In this case, better sleeping habits will develop with age.

Do not blame yourself for having a baby who does not sleep through the night or does not have a regular routine. It does not mean that you have failed because your baby does not have the same sleeping habits as other babies. Well-meaning friends and relatives can sometimes cause needless anxiety if they have expectations of ideal textbook behaviour to which your baby does not conform. Ultimately you and your family will develop your own routines which suit you and your lifestyle. These will possibly be quite different to the experiences of others.

During the early days with your new baby at home you may have to develop strategies to accommodate the changes in your life and to compensate for your disturbed sleep. You may have to make allowances in your daily activities. Some suggestions might include:

- Rest during the day whenever possible. If you have only one child, do this while he or she is sleeping. If you have other children, rest during their rest time.

- If you are struggling because of serious lack of sleep, ask for help from friends, relatives or neighbours. Perhaps offer to mind their children for a couple of hours, and while the favour is being reciprocated, you can catch up on some sleep.
- Your partner or husband could take the children for a picnic or to the park, leaving the house quiet for you to rest.

When putting your baby to bed for the night, ensure that the room is warm and that the baby is not hungry, is snugly and securely wrapped, and the nappy is dry. The baby needs to be warm, but not too hot. Always check that the wakefulness is not caused by some more serious problem such as colic, teething, infection or any other complaint. Teething may start any time after three months of age, but more usually around six months. These problems need to be dealt with using appropriate measures given elsewhere in this chapter. Regularly check the baby's weight through your local Maternal and Child Welfare Centre to ensure that the wakefulness is not caused by insufficient nourishment. Trust your intuition about whether there is some serious problem which needs to be investigated further.

If you are satisfied that there is no serious reason for the wakefulness, there are a number of things you can do to encourage more civilised sleeping habits. Babies are used to noise in the womb, your heartbeat and other body noises. Babies who come home from a noisy hospital environment may find it difficult to adjust to the quiet at home. Babies don't like silence or being left alone. A totally quiet environment may be unsettling. Some babies will sleep with soft, low music playing in the background. Other sounds which may help are the gentle ticking of a clock or the rhythmic bubbling of an aquarium. Played very softly, tapes of lullabies, of dolphin sounds or the sound of the sea can be very soothing. Make tapes of your own voice and the voices of other family members talking, telling stories or singing. Remember that babies respond to sounds with which they were familiar in the womb, so these sounds will be comforting and encourage sleep.

Encourage appropriate day and night behaviour. Babies do not know the difference between day and night, so it is important to establish a routine that involves play and wake time during the day and more emphasis on sleep at night. If the baby sleeps beautifully during the day, there will be less need to sleep well at night, so the aim would be to encourage less daytime sleep and more night-time sleep. Bath the baby at night as baths are very relaxing and encourage sleep. Chamomile in the bath water is very relaxing. Babies will usually sleep very well after the feed they have following bath time. Massage at bedtime is also relaxing and soothing. Use a massage oil blend with some lavender for extra relaxation. Night-time sleep should be in darkness, and daytime sleep with some filtered light in the room. This helps to adjust the baby's body clock to regular day and night sleeping behaviour. Don't keep the house quiet during the day. Allow the usual household noises during the day and use the soft, quiet sounds you have chosen for night-time.

Bach flowers such as Rescue Remedy may help if there is a change in routine or fear of being left alone. Other Bach flower remedies may also be suitable, for example, Aspen, Walnut, Chicory or Heather. Homoeopathic calming remedies are available from health food stores. These are often very helpful in breaking the cycle of wakefulness at night. Cranial osteopathy has helped many restless babies sleep well during the night.

If you are breastfeeding, do not drink coffee or tea late in the day. Coffee is stimulating and tea acts as a diuretic, which may reduce your milk supply during the evening. This might have the effect of causing the baby to wake earlier than if a plentiful supply of milk is available at the last feed of the day. Mothers breastfeeding babies with no dairy allergies can have a drink of warm milk about one hour before the last feed of the day.

Some babies will go off to sleep happily if being rocked, nursed or driven around in the family car. While some will stay asleep once put to bed, many wake the instant the motion is stopped. A very restless and demanding baby may be exhibiting early signs of hyperactivity. If this is the case, checking for possible allergens may help identify a trigger for these bouts of hyperactivity. Also, increase essential fatty acids in your diet if you are breastfeeding or, if you are not, ensure that the milk formula you use is enriched with them. You may have a child who is easily bored and needs a lot of attention and stimulation. If this is the case, encourage play and activity during daylight hours as much as possible. Carrying a restless baby in a sling during the day or evening may be soothing. Talk to your baby as you go about your daily tasks. This would keep him content and occupied.

Some people find that sleeping with the baby solves many problems. While some people are not comfortable with the idea and many believe that it may be a dangerous practice, there does not seem to be conclusive proof supporting this belief. Mothers in many indigenous societies sleep with their babies and they have few problems. If you decide that this is right for you, there are some benefits. The baby will feed as often as needed without disturbing you. You will get plenty of unbroken sleep, which can be a great advantage, especially if you have other children. If you decide to have your baby with you at night, you need a firm supporting bed rather than a soft mattress to ensure that your baby is safe while you sleep. Have the baby in the crook of your arm so that you will not roll onto him during the night. You may prefer to have the baby between you and the wall rather than between two adults in the bed, but make sure that there is no gap between the bed and the wall. Start the night with the baby in his own bed. As he gets older, the periods that he spends in his own bed will gradually get longer. You will gradually be able to encourage this as the child matures. Some older children will still come into their parents' bed occasionally if they are frightened or unable to sleep, but increasingly they will be able to respond to reassurance and a calming word from a parent.

Having your baby with you in bed will not spoil him. Babies need to be with their mother; fulfilling a need is not the same as spoiling.

If all else fails, some hospitals and birthing centres have mother and baby centres where you and your baby can learn to manage sleep behaviours. Many of these centres base their treatment on the premise that if the baby's food and comfort needs are met, then controlled crying will teach the baby that you will not attend to unnecessary crying. These centres also look after the baby while you catch up on much needed sleep. Just having this break from interrupted nights can be a welcome relief for a tired and frustrated mother. Some centres teach you techniques to encourage more appropriate day and night-time behaviour patterns in your baby. Ask your maternal and child health care nurse for the centre nearest to you.

Thrush

Thrush is quite common in infancy. It is caused by a fungus called candida albicans. In small numbers, it is a normal inhabitant of the intestines but it may proliferate, leading to an imbalance in the numbers of friendly bacteria which we need for digestion. This can happen after antibiotic use or if the immune system is overtaxed. It is common whenever there are allergies. Creamy white patches in the mouth over reddened areas suggest oral thrush. Thrush is sometimes a cause of nappy rash.

Thrush in an adult requires taking the probiotics called lactobacillus acidophilus and bifidus. If your baby has thrush, it is worth having a course of probiotics yourself. Take one teaspoon of an acidophilus and bifidus powder in water or two capsules twenty minutes before each meal. The flora of a baby's intestines is different to an adult's and requires a different probiotic. Babies and young children up to seven years of age need bifidobacterium infantis. Give this to your baby and take it yourself, as pregnant and lactating women will benefit their babies by using this probiotic.

If thrush is suspected, avoid all sugary foods and alcohol. Eat sourdough bread, as this will help you to avoid the yeast in normal bread. Also avoid mushrooms, vegemite and any fermented foods.

Homoeopathic remedies for candida can be used by both mother and baby.

Umbilical Cord

For a few days after the birth you will need to clean the umbilical cord until it drops off. Essential oil of cloves is a powerful antiseptic, and was used in the past to sterilise surgical instruments. It must not be used neat but diluted with water, use one drop only. Apply carefully with a piece of gauze. Diluted echinacea liquid can also be used in the same way.

Chapter 9

THE BACH FLOWER REMEDIES

Pregnancy, childbirth and new motherhood often bring huge emotional changes as a result of hormonal influences. The practical implications of enlarging a family will also bring challenges, frustrations and delights. Pregnant women are often very introspective and highly intuitive. In their heightened emotional state, pregnant women (and new mothers, too) often respond well to the gentle healing properties of flower remedies. These can be used during pregnancy to help calm fears, to gain confidence and to bring strength and serenity. During and after the birth they are calming, soothing and relaxing. Babies are often very responsive to flower remedies and their use early in a child's life can bring peace and harmony.

The Bach flower remedies can be used safely by anyone. The flower remedies have many uses during pregnancy and labour and some have been recommended for specific conditions in the relevant chapters in this book. There are others, however, which may suit you, your baby or other members of your family at other times in your life. For this reason this chapter describes each Bach flower remedy to give you an understanding of its actions and to enable you to choose remedies appropriate to your unique circumstances at any time in your life.

HISTORY OF THE BACH FLOWERS

During the 1930s, an English physician, Dr Edward Bach, became dissatisfied with the results obtained in his Harley Street medical practice. He turned to nature and wild flowers for a safe, simple and natural method of healing to restore vitality to the sick. Dr Bach believed that people's state of mind had a great impact on their health. This belief that psychological conditions could affect our physical health represented an enormous change in the thinking of the time.

Dr Bach believed that by prescribing according to moods or states of mind it would be possible to bring a feeling of peace and inner harmony, resulting in better health. He therefore set out to discover remedies to overcome negative emotional states and moods. The flower remedies he discovered in the English countryside are gentle, are not habit forming or harmful, have no side effects and will not interfere with any other treatment.

The Bach flower remedies are not a substitute for appropriate treatment of serious complaints. Rather, they help to support and strengthen the patient by dealing with the negative emotions which Dr Bach believed formed the basis of all disease.

There are thirty-eight Bach flower remedies covering several common negative states of mind. Dr Bach classified these remedies into seven categories: Fear, Oversensitivity, Uncertainty, Overcare for Others' Welfare, Loneliness, Insufficient Interest in Present Circumstances, and Despondency and Despair.

As you read through the description of each of the remedies, you will notice that the descriptions are often of quite extreme states of mind and represent the utmost emotional state for the remedy. It is possible to benefit from the use of the flower remedy even if your symptoms or thoughts are not as profound or extreme as the description suggests. As long as the general feeling or essence of the flower remedy matches your moods or emotions, you will benefit from its use.

You will also notice that both positive and negative aspects of the remedies' emotional states are given. This is because any negative state has a positive side to it. Dr Bach believed that to overcome a negative emotion it is important to do two things. First, recognise and acknowledge the fault. Second, and perhaps more important, develop the opposite virtue. This involves the concept of positive thinking, which he believed is much more powerful than focussing on negative aspects of our personalities. Anger, when used productively, can underlie our passion to seek change. Doubts about our abilities may challenge us and give us the impetus to understand our weaknesses and strengths, and to continue to improve ourselves. Feelings of guilt may be analysed to understand the concept of self-responsibility.

The positive aspects of the remedies represent the admirable human qualities of which we can be proud, the characteristics which bring us closer to our God-like nature. These include qualities such as courage, endurance, compassion, heroism, tolerance, honesty, loyalty, sympathy and love.

While reading about each remedy, read the first description, which may be quite negative. Then focus on the positive aspect. Note how that feels to you and whether it is a worthwhile and appropriate pursuit or change in your attitude. Some of the remedies give examples of people who may have exhibited these positive qualities. They are merely suggestions to encourage you and to give you some sense of and feel for the remedy. Please feel free to disagree and to find your own examples. You may also have some personal heroes who exemplify these qualities to you.

The affirmations are also there to help you. Use them as guidelines only. It may be more useful to formulate your own as you will develop affirmations that are highly personal and appropriate for you. Contemplate your affirmation regularly and use the flower remedies to support the changes you desire.

Some of the remedies have been marked with an asterisk. These remedies may be used in a couple of different ways. They can be used for emotions that correspond to a person's type or constitution. For example, Beech is for the critical person who always finds fault with everyone and everything and is never satisfied. But the remedies may also correspond to temporary circumstances. Even the most sweet natured and tolerant of us may occasionally find ourselves temporarily bothered by the annoying habits or idiosyncrasies of others.

Beech is also appropriate in this instance. In the former case, the remedy may need to be given for a long period of time to affect a deep change, while in the latter case it may need to be given only occasionally as the need arises.

When using the Bach flower remedies, it is important to keep in mind that they will help and support your other treatments. Never try to deal with serious conditions without proper professional support.

FEAR

Rock Rose

Keywords: Absolute terror, panic
Used in grave situations where there is extreme fear, for example, nightmares and panic attacks.
Positive: Heroism
Feats of heroism in the face of great fear illustrate the wonderful positive side of Rock Rose. They demonstrate the great heights to which humans can aspire.
Affirmation: I have faith in my strength to overcome any obstacles.

Mimulus *

Keywords: Fear with a known cause
Mimulus has less extreme fear than the absolute terror of Rock Rose. However, any fear can paralyse us and prevent us from reaching our potential. There is always a known reason for the Mimulus fear, although the fear may be quite irrational.
People whose constitutional type is Mimulus tend to be shy and nervous, like the child who hides behind his mother's skirts when there is no real threat or danger.
Positive: Understanding and courage to face life's trials.
The courage to face our fears and the recognition that they can have control over us only if we allow them to are very powerful and liberating.

Affirmation: I acknowledge my fear and understand that it has no power to prevent me from continuing to pursue my dreams.

Cherry Plum

Keywords: Fear of losing one's mind, despair, deep depression

Cherry Plum has very great desperation and is a serious and extreme condition. May feel on the verge of a nervous breakdown or of being out of control.

Positive: Calmness and courage in the face of adversity. To acknowledge and overcome these strong and destructive emotions requires great commitment and courage, but is a powerful step on the road to healing. Nelson Mandela may have experienced this great despair during his incarceration. However, he emerged full of confidence in the rightness of his cause.

Affirmation: I trust in a higher purpose for my suffering and have faith that there is something better for me.

Aspen

Keywords: Inexplicable, groundless fear

Unlike Mimulus, where the object of the fear is known, the Aspen fear does not know its cause and may be vague and amorphous. Alternatively, the fear may appear groundless and illogical. Nervousness, sudden unaccountable fears, goose bumps or a feeling that it is all in the imagination may suggest a need for Aspen. The fear may be accompanied by uncontrollable shaking, sweating and panic attacks. Dr Bach believed that fear of the Aspen type is often connected with thoughts of death or religion.

Positive: Courage and the desire to experience adventure and novel situations.

Pioneers show us the positive aspect of Aspen. Some may have crossed physical barriers such as the ocean, a continent or the heavens. Others challenged the boundaries of contemporary understanding and beliefs. In their search for a better life or greater knowledge they demonstrate our human thirst for awareness and a constant desire to push aside the limits and boundaries of our world.

Affirmation: I strive towards my goal. My fear will help me recognise the path and I know I have the strength to follow it.

Red Chestnut*

Keywords: Excessive fear for others

This is the person who worries excessively for others, usually for children or for very close friends or relatives. This worry may become obsessive and stifle the object of the concern. The worrier always anticipates trouble and expects that the worst will happen. This is normal love taken to a debilitating extreme. The overprotective mother, always anxious for her child's safety, may not allow the child some freedom to find his own boundaries. This often continues into the child's adulthood, and is a classic example of the Red Chestnut type.

Positive: Offering strength and support for others in emergencies.

Mary, Mother of Jesus, showed great love for her son, but always gave him the freedom to follow His own path.

Affirmation: I love and cherish and watch over you. I give you the freedom to find your own path in life and to walk it with my blessing.

UNCERTAINTY

Cerato *

Keywords: Self-doubts

Lacking the courage of their convictions, Cerato people continually seek the opinions of others and might even compromise their own beliefs to follow the advice of others. Although often very capable, their own doubts, uncertainties and misgivings cause the Cerato people to be followers rather than to strike out in their own direction.

Positive: Self-assurance and personal integrity.

Joan of Arc suffered great hardship and a painful death to follow her dreams and her beliefs, in spite of the fact that she was only a young girl in a male dominated society, ridiculed and scorned by many.

Affirmation: I have trust and faith in my convictions and my integrity. I respect the opinion of others, but choose my own beliefs.

Scleranthus *

Keywords: Uncertainty, indecision

The Scleranthus state of mind is indecisive, alternating between two choices. This may involve choosing between two courses of action or it may manifest on the emotional plane, resulting in moodiness and swings of emotion, such as alternating happiness and sadness, talkativeness or silence, laughing or crying, or erratic and rambling conversation. This lack of centredness may manifest as erratic symptoms and wandering aches and pains. Out-of-kilter Librans who have not developed the typical balance of this star sign may be all over the place in their thoughts and their behaviours, demonstrating the Scleranthus indecisiveness. The Scleranthus person, although indecisive, does not ask advice of others the way Cerato does.

Positive: Confidence and self-assurance to rely on one's own good judgement.

Firefighters display the positive aspects of Scleranthus. They rely on their experience and judgement to choose their course of action, and then act quickly and decisively.

Affirmation: I choose my course of action in full recognition of the facts and trusting that there are many valid paths to the same end.

Gentian *

Keywords: Self-doubt, discouragement

A negative outlook leads to easy discouragement when things go wrong. Gentian is valuable for people with a negative approach to everything they attempt; they almost fail before they have even started. It is also useful for anyone who experiences a temporary setback in his or her plans. This may happen to any of us and Gentian may give us the strength to persevere and not give up. For example, think of Gentian for the unemployed when searching for a job, or for students discouraged by poor performance in exams.

Positive: Courage to persevere and to do one's best.

Affirmation: Every day I move a little closer to my goal.

Gorse

Keywords: Disappointment, despair

After repeated failures or disappointments, the feeling that it is useless to keep trying suggests a need for Gorse. Gorse is generally more extreme than Gentian in that failures have occurred more often. It is of value in any situation where there has been little progress despite repeated efforts. For example, it is useful at the start of any long project or during a long illness to give the strength to persist despite the ups and downs which are bound to occur along the way.

A worn or haggard appearance, perhaps with dark circles under the eyes, suggests repeated failures and disappointments and therefore a need for Gorse.

Positive: Belief in oneself and in the light at the end of the tunnel.

The drug-dependent person who strives to overcome his addiction in spite of many difficulties and setbacks shows the positive Gorse qualities. Giving up smoking can be a very Gorse-like experience: the going often gets tougher the longer you are into the non-smoking program. Often many people give up several times before they can finally give the habit away permanently.

Affirmation: Each attempt gives me a better understanding of myself and the importance of striving towards my goal.

Hornbeam

Keywords: Physical and mental fatigue
Lack of energy and insufficient strength to get through the day make coping with mundane and routine matters difficult. If you find that you can be motivated by some new or thrilling project, but do not have the strength for more everyday concerns, then Hornbeam may be what you need. The tiredness of Hornbeam is generally less complete and overwhelming than that of Olive.
Positive: Stamina to cope with life, its joys and its ups and downs.
Affirmation: I enjoy my life and I allow myself both busy and quiet times.

Wild Oat

Keywords: Career indecision
Wild Oat is useful for talented, ambitious people who may need to choose between various viable career possibilities. There may be many different avenues for us to achieve and realise our full potential. Wild Oat will help us to find a career and to be satisfied and fulfilled with our choice.Alternatively, unfulfilled ambition or finding oneself frustrated and bored in an unsuitable and unfulfilling work environment may be helped by Wild Oat. It may help us find and work towards our true path in life.
Think of Wild Oat for students struggling with career choices or for anyone considering a career change.
Wild Oat is sometimes good if many remedies are indicated, or if it is difficult to select a remedy. (Holly is another good remedy to think of if you can't find the best one to start with.)
Positive: Clear ambitions, fulfilling one's purpose in life.

Affirmation: I am working in my ideal career and following my goals and my dreams.

INSUFFICIENT INTEREST IN PRESENT CIRCUMSTANCES

Clematis *

Keywords: Daydreaming, vagueness

Withdrawal into a private fantasy world to avoid unpleasantness can be an escape from reality and a refusal to deal with problems. Preoccupation, absent-mindedness and the vacant, far-away look of people who prefer to be alone with their thoughts may respond to Clematis. Heavy sleepers and those who struggle to wake from sleep may also respond to the remedy.

Temporary vagueness can be felt by any of us when feeling faint, or after the shock of receiving bad news. If this vague or unreal state continues after its use as a defence mechanism, then Clematis may help the person to gently come back to acknowledge the present.

Positive: Alert, creative and open to inspiration.

Idealists, many mystics and those who meditate exhibit the positive aspect of Clematis, as do artists with their creative use of their introspective skills. Prayer, which takes us to thoughts of higher ideals, is also a useful application of the Clematis state.

Affirmation: I am interested in everyone and everything about me. I bring the strength I gain from my introspective times to enhance my joy in being with others.

Honeysuckle

Keywords: Nostalgia, homesickness

While it is important to learn from our past and to use our experiences to live fulfilling lives, we should not dwell on the past to the exclusion of the present. A life spent brooding in sadness or fear or longing for the past misses the opportunity to experience the joys of the present and the chance to adapt the lessons from the past to enrich the present. People who long for 'the good old days' or migrants who do not adapt but constantly make unhappy comparisons with their old life miss the opportunity for new joys and experiences.

Positive: Use the experiences of the past to enrich life in the present.

Migrants who settle in a new land, bringing the richness of their culture while also immersing themselves in the new, demonstrate the positive power of Honeysuckle. They are able to adapt their knowledge to enrich their own lives and the new country they have settled.

Affirmation: I welcome and enjoy new experiences. I remember and release past memories and bring their blessings into my new life.

Wild Rose

Keywords: Resignation, apathy

Apathy and lack of interest is a typical Wild Rose state. Resignation to an unhappy state or an illness will not inspire us to pursue our goals or ambitions. If we fail to make any effort to change our circumstances, then the low vitality, monotony and boredom will become self-perpetuating. A need for Wild Rose may be manifested as an expressionless drone to the voice or expressionless demeanour.

Positive: Vitality, purpose

Edward 'Weary' Dunlop showed the positive aspect of Wild Rose in refusing to give in to the depression and misery of life in a POW camp. He inspired others with his will to survive and help those he lived with.

Affirmation: I am constantly delighted by the richness of life and the many new experiences I can enjoy.

Olive

Keywords: Complete mental and physical exhaustion
The fatigue of Olive is complete and overwhelming. The mind and the body feel totally drained, and there are no reserves of energy left to draw on. This may occur after long periods of stress or illness, or in people who lead lives so busy and full that they have no time for relaxation.

Quiet times, holidays and relaxation need to be a regular part of our lives. During these times we replenish our depleted energy stores, restore our interest in life and break from our daily routine. If we do not allow ourselves these important times, we are at risk of experiencing the extreme tiredness of the Olive state. This is especially true in the current work climate, where many people are working unrealistically long hours.

Give Olive during a long convalescence or during stressful and demanding times to maintain the body's strength. Olive can encourage people to benefit from rest and to revitalise their body, mind and spirit.

Positive: Strength and stamina when needed, ability to restore reserves when resting.

Affirmation: I enjoy the fullness of my life, but regularly allow myself the time and space to relax and to just be.

White Chestnut

Keywords: Constant mental arguments, continual negative thoughts
When we go over and over the same situation with thoughts that circulate in our head without resolution, preoccupation with past wrongs can result in depression and fatigue and take away our zest for fully experiencing the present. This constant war being waged in our mind may be a cause of insomnia, lack of focus on the present, or difficulty in concentrating.

Positive: Let the past go and know that you did the best you could at the time.

The tenacity of White Chestnut is reflected in loyalty to a person or a cause. Persistence and determination to work unceasingly towards a goal also demonstrate the positive aspect of White Chestnut.

Affirmation: I release old wounds and hurts. I strive willingly and happily towards my new goal.

Mustard

Keywords: Sudden, black depression with no known cause

When deep despair descends suddenly for no obvious reason and some time later lifts just as inexplicably, think of Mustard. During this time of black depression, nothing seems to bring any comfort and nothing seems worthwhile. Mustard can be given during the episodes of despair. It is also appropriate to use Mustard between episodes to reduce the tendency to these inexplicable fits of depression.

Positive: Calmness, peace of mind

Affirmation: I am in control of my thoughts and I choose to see the positives in my life.

Chestnut Bud

Keywords: Failure to learn from experience, constantly repeats mistakes

Inability to learn from past mistakes and to link consequences with actions leads to these mistakes being repeated constantly. The pet that keeps soiling inside the house despite the unpleasant consequences, the woman who seeks the same unsuitable characteristics in each of her partners, and the person who often has accidents or mishaps have not learnt the lessons behind their actions. Whether this appears to be due to impatience, disinterest, or lack of concentration, think of Chestnut Bud. There may also possibly be awkwardness and clumsiness if this remedy is needed, as the person is not fully concentrating on his circumstances and has not learnt to control his movements.

Positive: Maintains attention, focussed to learn easily.
Affirmation: I learn easily and eagerly from all life's lessons. I aspire to new and exciting tasks and experiences.

LONELINESS

Water Violet *

Keywords: Proud, aloof
Quiet, gentle and self-reliant people may prefer their own company when ill or distressed. This describes the Water Violet person who may find it difficult to communicate his thoughts and feelings to others.
Water Violet people may appear arrogant and condescending. This, however, may be because of their inherent shyness and not because of any sense of superiority. Some may feel that they are a little different to others, although they would not admit this. Physically, these tendencies may manifest as tense and tight muscles.
Positive: Serene, sympathetic and dignified.
Affirmation: I relax with myself and with my trusted friends. My wisdom and my quiet dignity are often needed by others in their search for peace.

Impatiens *

Keywords: Impatience and irritability
Impatiens, as the name suggests, is for any state where there is impatience and a sense of hurry or urgency. Impatiens people move quickly and may exhaust themselves through frustration and nervousness. Always rushing about, they may be quite accident prone as they are in too much of a hurry to take care and to watch where they are going. The Impatiens type is subject to pain caused by sudden cramps and spasms.
Positive: Motivated, capable and patient.
Michelangelo demonstrated endless patience in his detailed work on the ceiling of the Sistine Chapel. His attention to

detail was stunning, but he never lost sight of his overall goals.
Affirmation: I am able to concentrate on fine detail while keeping in mind the bigger picture.

Heather *

Keywords: Self-centred, worries about oneself
People who constantly discuss their difficulties and illnesses have a genuine need to be understood and appreciated, but unfortunately their incessant talk only serves to drive others away. At their worst, these people will stand very close to you, allowing you no escape. They must be the centre of attention. These are often the so-called hypochondriacs who have always had the most dreadful experience, much worse than anyone else's, the worst case ever seen and so on. They are unhappy by themselves, but are unable to listen to anyone else's problems.
Positive: Understanding through personal suffering, compassionate.
Many counsellors demonstrate the positive aspect of Heather. They will listen and advise, and will draw on their expertise and their previous experiences to help the person who seeks their assistance. Their own problems are never used for sympathy or attention.
Affirmation: I recognise that I am worthy of great love and understanding. I use my powerful understanding of suffering and sorrow to help others overcome the sadness in their lives.

OVERSENSITIVITY

Agrimony *

Keywords: Worry but with a cheerful and happy-go-lucky appearance
It is a pleasure to be with these happy and carefree people. They have a good sense of humour, and hate any arguments or signs of divisiveness or enmity between people. When in dis-

tress, they seek company to help them forget their problems, but not to constantly bemoan their fate as Heather may do. They will make light of their sufferings, and may use drugs or alcohol to temporarily deaden the pain. However, they may be restless at night or when they are alone, going over and over their thoughts. The mask of a clown is often said to hide much pain and suffering.

Positive: Optimism, comedians

Affirmation: I have close friends I can trust with my deepest worries and concerns. I enjoy good company and share much joy and laughter with my friends.

Centaury *

Keywords: Submissive, timid

Easily dominated and weak-willed, Centaury people will obey more dominating people. They may constantly do favours for others against their own wishes and needs. They may be tied to demanding parents and unable to exercise their right to choose their own path in life. For example, they may follow their parents' choice of career when it is not really what they want, or they may allow their parents to dictate their choice of spouse instead of following their heart. They often appear pale, submissive and tired. Centaury may give them the strength to stand up for their beliefs and the courage to make their own choices. It may also be useful after a long illness when there is lack of vitality and determination to recover.

Positive: Strength to follow one's own beliefs and one's own path in life.

Ability to help others with dignity and respect, but only in the best interests of both giver and receiver. Volunteer work, when done with quiet humility for the wellbeing of others, indicates the sense of service which Centaury may develop. Volunteers who never lose their own identity and never make their personal needs subservient to the needs of others are the Centaury type.

Affirmation: I stand in my own integrity and live my life according to principles of personal responsibility. I help and care for others with the same honesty and accountability.

Walnut

Keywords: Major life change, change in thought patterns and habits

Walnut helps to break with the old and establish the new. Ties to any old habits or restrictions which no longer serve us and need to be replaced can be broken with the help of Walnut. It is useful for any time of change such as during teething, puberty, menopause, change of religion, change of occupation or migration to another country.

Positive: Independence, pioneering spirit, welcoming new ideas and new experiences.

Dr Bach exemplified the Walnut type. He turned his back on conventional ideas of medicine to develop a way which he felt was more in tune with his ideas of health and healing.

Affirmation: I welcome new and exciting experiences. I integrate new and old experiences to enrich my own life and the lives of others.

Holly

Keywords: Jealousy, bitterness, hatred, any strong negative emotional state

Holly covers any strong negative emotion whether it be jealousy, envy, bitterness or resentment. These negative emotions may be well below the surface and it is often difficult to recognise them, especially in ourselves.

Holly is extremely useful if many remedies seem to be indicated and no single remedy stands out as being more needed than any others. It may help to clear any underlying negative tendencies which may be at the root of the presenting problem. (Another remedy to consider if many are indicated is Wild Oat.)

Positive: Genuine happiness for the good fortunes of others, personal satisfaction.

Affirmation: I enjoy my life and my friends. I share my successes with them as they share theirs with me. Happiness and success for any of us is a source of great joy and pride to me.

DESPONDENCY AND DESPAIR

Larch *

Keywords: Low self-confidence, inferiority complex
The Larch type is self-effacing, suffering false modesty. Larch type people seldom attempt anything because they think they will fail. They are easily discouraged and are great procrastinators. They are not frightened like Mimulus and, unlike Holly, they are not envious of the success of others. Larch may be associated with some cases of impotence.
Positive: Eagerness for new experiences, self-confidence.
In the later years of her life, Princess Diana showed some Larch characteristics in continuing her charity work despite her inherent modesty. Earlier in her life, she possibly exhibited more Mimulus and Gentian or Gorse qualities.
Affirmation: I welcome new experiences and new friends. I trust my innate good sense to protect and guide me.

Pine

Keywords: Feelings of guilt
Pine people will dwell on their mistakes, feeling guilt and disappointment with themselves. Often they are perfectionists who set unrealistically high standards for themselves. These expectations inevitably lead to guilt as they cannot always be fulfilled. Pine may also take on responsibility for the mistakes and faults of others. As a result of these feelings of guilt and inadequacy, Pine people may overwork in their effort to prove themselves, and become easily tired and depressed.
Positive: Accurate perception of personal responsibility and willingness to learn from mistakes.

Affirmation: I accept responsibility for my mistakes, accepting that I always do my best. I am always honest in my thoughts and my behaviour, and always do my utmost to live to my perfect ideals.

Elm*

Keywords: Great responsibility, temporary self-doubts
The Elm type is highly competent and generally confident. Elm types are often in extremely responsible positions requiring great skill and proficiency. Their profession may involve service of some kind such as caring for others in the healing, counselling or teaching professions. They know that they have chosen their vocation wisely and that they have the ability to do the job well. At times they may become overwhelmed by temporary feelings of inadequacy, resulting in exhaustion and doubts about their abilities. It is at times like these that Elm may give them the strength to persevere and overcome any obstacles to continuing their good work.
Positive: Self-confidence and trust in their great abilities.
Many teachers and nurses have the Elm characteristics of quietly doing great work in their chosen profession, despite the often overwhelming and thankless nature of the task.
Affirmation: I am strong and capable. I enjoy and value my work. I allow myself time for rest and relaxation to revitalise my body and my mind.

Sweet Chestnut

Keywords: Extreme despair, hopelessness
Sweet Chestnut is for those times referred to as 'the dark night of the soul'. If Sweet Chestnut is needed, the limits of human endurance have been passed. There is a feeling that there is no hope, no future and no end to the despair. Like Cherry Plum, this is an extreme condition which would require professional help.

Positive: Trust in a higher purpose for our existence; the compassion to help others through their 'dark night'.
Jesus Christ would have experienced this total despair during the last days of his life. However, He always trusted in the love of His Father and knew that He was following His true path for a greater good.
Affirmation: I trust that God will look after me and bring me to safety.

Star of Bethlehem

Keyword: Shock
Used for any shock such as sudden bad news, a fright, or an accident. The effects of shock may be immediate or delayed, but there will often be a lasting effect, even long after the incident has been forgotten. Star of Bethlehem is often needed as an aid in the treatment of stomach ulcers. By removing the memory of underlying trauma, Star of Bethlehem may be a catalyst for other remedies to work. Use for both mother and child after birth.
Positive: The presence of mind and the courage to stay focussed in the present and to act appropriately in any crisis.
Affirmation: I have the courage and strength to deal with this situation.

Willow*

Keywords: Resentment and bitterness, apportions blame
The Willow feeling is one of having been unfairly and undeservedly chosen to suffer. Self-centred and self-pitying people who complain, are never satisfied and bear grudges may benefit from Willow. They will always be able to find some misery in their lives and are generally uninterested in the problems of others, except to compare their own fate with another's good fortune. They will blame everyone but themselves for their plight. This is the exact opposite of Pine, who will take on the guilt and responsibility for everyone's problems, including their own.

Any of us can lose our sense of perspective temporarily and feel that we have been badly done by. Willow will help us regain our good sense and optimism.

Positive: Acceptance of personal responsibility for our thoughts and actions.

Positive Willow might be seen in the writings of Anne Frank, who described her time in the concentration camp with such clarity, but without bitterness or rancour.

Affirmation: I accept responsibility for my thoughts. I willingly share the highs and the lows in the lives of my friends.

Oak *

Keywords: Strain after great efforts and feats of endurance

Strong, capable and reliable people who often work long hours and take on enormous responsibilities may find that these long hours of overwork lead to great stress and the possibility of breakdown. With Oak these strong and capable people may find the strength to continue.

Positive: Courage to continue in spite of great hardship.

Mother Theresa continued to bring help to the poor well into her old age and illness. She quietly pursued her goals in spite of the long hours of work and the numerous difficulties and hardships involved.

Affirmation: I believe in myself and the goodness of my task. I have the strength and courage to persevere, and I am able to rely on others to share my load.

Crab Apple

Keyword: Cleansing remedy

Crab Apple is the cleansing remedy. This cleansing may apply to a physical or an emotional condition. For example, physical conditions may be discharges or skin problems. Emotional conditions might include a bad habit or an obsession with appearances. With any of these conditions, Crab Apple will cleanse the mind of the feeling of uncleanliness that accompanies the physical or emotional manifestation.

Positive: Understanding that a physical problem is a manifestation of a deeper, internal disorder.

Affirmation: I release any negative thoughts I have about myself. I am able to honour and respect myself.

OVERCARE FOR THE WELFARE OF OTHERS

Chicory *

Keywords: Possessive, demanding
Chicory is for those times when we feel the need to control and direct the lives of others. Instead of giving love we may wish to possess and control. The Chicory type people demand respect and unquestioning obedience to their wishes. They cannot appreciate that the only respect that is worth having is the respect that has been earned through personal integrity. They also need to learn to respect the wishes of others and to understand that these wishes have validity. Chicory is useful for very demanding children or for the possessive mother unable to allow her children the freedom to lead their own lives in their own way. Centaury, with its submissiveness, may easily become prey to the Chicory demand for obedience.

Positive: Unselfish nurturing and care for others.

Affirmation: I love and care for you. I respect your wishes and your right to choose your destiny.

Vervain *

Keyword: Over-enthusiasm and fanaticism
Fanatics and zealots hold strong opinions, and are sometimes so caught up in the importance of their cause that they find it difficult to accept that others do not support their cause completely. They need to develop a little patience and understanding, which Vervain may help them achieve. These people are often highly strung and may live on their nerves, finding it dif-

ficult to sleep or relax. Tension, headaches, eye strain and muscular spasms may result from their devoted attention to their task.

Positive: Calmness and the wisdom to make a valuable contribution, tempered by respect for the beliefs of others.

The Dalai Lama may represent the positive aspect of Vervain. While devoted to the correctness of his cause, he approaches the political and religious tasks of his office with calmness and patience.

Dr Bach himself was a Vervain with a devotion to his chosen task and an unswerving belief in the rightness of it. While making the remedies available to all, he also respected people's rights to come to the remedies in their own time.

Affirmation: I am confident and sure in my beliefs, and I will strive honestly to achieve whatever goals this brings. At all times I respect your right to choose your own opinions and your own goals.

Vine *

Keywords: Domineering, ruthless, efficient

Vine people are highly efficient; they are born leaders and are generally in positions of authority. As strong leaders and rulers they generally expect and receive unquestioning loyalty and obedience. While their strong vision of leadership may lead them to make decisions which are economically and politically expedient, these decisions may be morally or ethically deficient. Dictators represent the extreme Vine character, with its ruthless demand for total obedience. The Vine's unyielding attitude may be reflected in headaches, high blood pressure, muscular tension and other complaints associated with rigidity and inflexibility.

Positive: Strength to rule wisely and justly with compassion.

Solomon and King David were powerful kings who ruled wisely for all their subjects.

Affirmation: I accept my talents and understand that they are to be used for the good of others, including my family and my friends.

Beech *

Keywords: Intolerance, criticism

Beech people constantly find fault with others. They cannot allow for individual differences or accept that there are many ways of doing things. They may be very lonely people as they crave acceptance, but push others away from them with their constant fault finding. The highly critical mother-in-law is the archetype of this remedy. At times, however, we may all exhibit Beech-type symptoms as, for example, when we find ourselves annoyed by the idiosyncrasies or habits of others.

Positive: Tolerance towards others and joy in the diversity of human qualities.

Jesus exhibited perfect tolerance in his love for all humankind, despite our many faults.

Affirmation: I celebrate and honour the diversity of talents, of cultures, and of opinions demonstrated by my friends and my family.

Rock Water

Keywords: Self-denial

These are people who are very hard on themselves. They may follow strict diets or regimens and be quite inflexible about their routines, unable to deviate from their ordered habits. They often have very strong opinions, especially about religion or politics. This is the only Bach flower remedy not made from plants; it reflects the strength and permanence of the rock, able to be worn away only by the sheer dogged persistence of running water.

Positive: Strong personal integrity

Mahatma Gandhi lived a life of poverty and was prepared to sacrifice his life for his beliefs and in his attempts to convince others of the truth of his message. He did this quietly and lovingly.

Affirmation: I pursue my goals with determination and persistence. However, I still allow myself to enjoy and appreciate the beautiful things in life: the smell of a rose, a beautiful landscape, a stirring piece of music, a great bottle of wine or a delicious meal.

Rescue Remedy

Rescue Remedy is, as the name suggests, for any feeling of crisis or emergency. It can be used frequently during childbirth, panic attacks or for the after-effects of any such state. It contains five flower remedies: Star of Bethlehem, for shock; Rock Rose, for terror and panic; Impatiens, for impatience and the sense of urgency and panic; Cherry Plum, for extreme despair and hopelessness; and Clematis, for vagueness.

PRESCRIBING A REMEDY

Flower remedies can be used in two ways. They can be used for an acute condition, in which case the remedy is often obvious. For example, this would be the case in any difficult or traumatic situation where Rescue Remedy is a necessary choice, or if you were feeling annoyed and needed some Beech.

Flower remedies can also be used for chronic conditions, in which case you need to follow the guidelines set out here to help you make your choice. These are guidelines only to get you thinking and to help you analyse your motives and your emotional responses to situations. Remember that you are looking for your own emotional responses to events in your life, not the way you think you should behave or the way that others might behave. You need to be honest. The feelings you need to know about are yours alone; they are entirely personal and subjective.

Think back over your life:

- As a child did you lack self-confidence or were you easily discouraged?
- Recall any traumatic incidents in your life. For example, did you ever change homes or schools? What was your response to these incidents?
- As an adult do you exhaust yourself by overwork or worry, or do you bury yourself in daydreaming?
- Was there some trauma or unpleasant episode in your life which has changed you dramatically?
- Are there any areas of your life that stand out as needing some special care? For example, are you easily irritated or do you get very impatient with the foibles of others?
- Have there been any particular psychological patterns or patterns of behaviour? Do you try to work things out by yourself without letting others know or do you tell everyone your problems? Do you seek and heed the advice of others?

Choose the remedies which match your personal history most closely. Limit the remedies to three or four if there is more than one that seems to be suitable. Go with your instincts if you are having trouble choosing.

Regularly focus on the positive aspect of the remedy and on any affirmations which you feel are appropriate. Think about the changes which you would like to develop in yourself. Reward yourself when you notice any improvement and change in your reactions to situations. Notice how this new reaction feels and what positive benefits there are in this new response. Visualise yourself repeating the new behaviour or reaction.

Don't worry if there are no immediate or dramatic changes. Sometimes you may experience a change overnight, but often changes are much slower, especially if the problem is deep-seated or of long standing. Habits that have been with us a long while may be resistant to change. The effects of the remedies may be quite subtle and deep acting. As the remedies have their effects and your feelings change, you may need to move to other remedies.

If there appears to be no change after a few weeks, other factors may be involved in your emotions and you may need to rethink and choose other remedies. Consider a course of Holly, Wild Oat or Star of Bethlehem to act as a catalyst. Then go through the same process as before to choose other remedies. Alternatively, see a practitioner who can advise you on Bach flower remedies. Rest assured, however, that if you have chosen the remedies incorrectly, there will be no ill effects.

You might recognise your family or friends or even your pets in many of the remedies. Feel free to prescribe for your young children or for your pets. They will not be able to repeat the affirmations, but will still benefit from the use of the remedies. Children and pets, and even plants, respond very well to the flower remedies. Their motives are often much closer to the surface than those of adults. Over many years we build on and perhaps even bury the earliest manifestations of our distress, making it much more difficult to unravel the many complicated layers.

Recommend the flower remedies to adults and older children only if they are willing and responsive. Respect others' right to choose their own path. If you find yourself becoming a crusader, consider Vervain for yourself!

Using the Remedies

Use no more than three or four remedies at any one time. They tend to work more effectively if you do not use too many at a time. (Rescue Remedy is an exception to this rule.)

Once you have chosen the required remedy or remedies, follow these steps:

- Take the flower remedy straight from the stock bottle.
- More economically, obtain a small, clean bottle, preferably one with a dropper. Add one teaspoon of brandy to act as a

preservative and fill with plain spring water or tap water. Add two drops of each of the chosen flower remedies. You will then be able to put the stock bottle away for further use later.

- Take four drops either directly on the tongue or in a drink at least four times a day.
- Repeat to yourself or write down the appropriate affirmation each time you take the remedy and first thing in the morning and last thing at night.

The flower remedies can be taken more frequently if needed, such as in a crisis situation or during panic attacks.

Continue taking the remedy for up to three weeks at a time. This allows some integration time. During this time your body will accept the new emotional response and incorporate it into your behaviour patterns. For example, after taking Gentian you may find that you respond less negatively to disappointments and are able to see setbacks as temporary problems only. You may realise that you do not always go looking for things that could go wrong, but are much more aware of the good things that are happening in your life. After this time, have a break for about a week. Either return to the original remedy combination or renew your choice.

In his book, *Heal Thyself - an explanation of the real cause and cure of disease*, Dr Bach demonstrates great love and compassion for the human condition and the difficulties we face in our daily lives. His flower remedies are a gift to bring us comfort, to support us on our path through life and to help us develop the great potential that is our human birthright.

There is no better way to conclude this chapter than by quoting Dr Bach, demonstrating his deep love of humanity and his recognition of the struggles we are faced with: ". . . the real victories of life come through love and gentleness . . ." And also:

But in the darkest hours, and when success seems well-nigh impossible, let us ever remember that God's children should never be afraid, that our Souls only give us such tasks as we are capable of accomplishing, and that with our own courage and faith in the Divinity within us victory must come to all who continue to strive.

Chapter 10

THE TISSUE SALTS

Pregnancy is a time of heightened nutritional requirements, with a huge demand placed on the mother by the growing foetus. There are also the demands of the pregnancy itself with the increase in the mother's blood supply and growth of the uterus and other tissue necessary for survival of the new life. It is often a time when difficulties with supply, absorption and assimilation of nutrients become more obvious. For example, cramps suggest an increased need for magnesium and tiredness may suggest greater need for iron. Some cravings suggest a need for certain nutrients. Lack of these needed nutrients causes the body to send out a cry for the missing substance. This cry may be experienced as an increased urge for foods which contain nutrients similar to those needed. The urge for pickles and ice cream may be an urge for calcium and some less well-known minerals such as potassium. Craving for beer may reflect an increased need for B vitamins, and an increased need for calories and carbohydrates might be suggested by craving for wine, fruit or cakes and biscuits.

The Schuessler tissue salts are a simple method of improving absorption and assimilation of various minerals. Some of the tissue salts have been recommended in earlier chapters to help with certain problems. This chapter describes all twelve of the tissue salts and gives you some insight into their use during and after pregnancy. You can, however, use them at any other time to help the absorption of the particular tissue salts that are needed and, therefore, to deal with many common problems simply and quickly.

The human body consists of a complex arrangement of water, organic substances and inorganic minerals. During the late nineteenth century, Dr Schuessler developed his ideas about the inorganic minerals found in the human body. He studied the twelve substances that are most prevalent in the human body and maintained that an imbalance in any of them could contribute to disease. He further postulated that correcting the imbalance would lead to improved health. By using very small doses of the minerals he could encourage the body to assimilate these same minerals more efficiently, thus contributing to balance and harmony in the body. He named these small doses of minerals 'tissue salts' in recognition of their role in nourishing the tissues of the body. The tissue salts, therefore, were developed to enable the body to absorb, assimilate and metabolise these vital minerals.

These minerals generally come from our foods. But while they may be present in adequate quantities in our diet, they can be of benefit only if we absorb and utilise them correctly. The tissue salts help with this absorption and assimilation. Being a vital part of the body, the tissue salts are not a drug; they are considered to be a food, and help with the assimilation of the food we eat.

As you read the descriptions of the tissue salts, notice the keyword or keywords which sum up the overall action of the tissue salt. Notice also the likes and dislikes of the tissue salt. When a person needs any particular tissue salt, you will also find that these likes or dislikes may be present. This can help you choose between different tissue salts if many seem to be suggested.

The following descriptions of the tissue salts are brief and are intended to give you only a feel for their action. For any serious problem, have your tissue salts chosen by a naturopath or a homoeopath. Tissue salts need to be considered carefully if you are taking any prescription drugs. For example, Silica will push a problem out of your system, whereas creams for rashes or antibiotics for acne suppress the inflammatory response. The tissue salt and the cream or antibiotic will oppose each other.

Calc Fluor (Calcium Fluoride)

Keywords: **Lack of elasticity and flexibility**
Preferences: **Likes heat**
               Hates weather changes

Calc Fluor is found in the bones, nails and teeth, in the walls of the blood vessels and in the skin. Lack of tissue elasticity suggests improper metabolism of Calc Fluor. In the bones, nails and teeth, this might be evident in broken bones that knit slowly, nails that split easily, or easy tooth decay. If the problem affects the blood vessels, there may be a tendency to haemorrhoids or varicose veins. In the skin, problems such as cysts and scars that don't heal or heal in hardened knots may benefit from the use of Calc Fluor.

Do not take Calc Fluor during pregnancy. With its toning and strengthening effect on tissue it may oppose the normal slackening effect of pregnancy hormones on ligaments which need to relax in preparation for childbirth. It is fine at any other time, including while breastfeeding. For haemorrhoids and varicose veins during pregnancy, use witch-hazel instead.

Calc Phos (Calcium Phosphate)

Keywords: **Nutrition tonic**
Preferences: **Likes warmth and dry weather**
               Hates damp and cold weather
               Hates changes in the weather

Calc Phos is found in the bones, teeth, blood and gastric juices. It is especially useful for problems or aches and pains in the skeletal system. These might be the growing pains of rapidly growing children or problems of calcium assimilation resulting in osteoporosis. It helps build strong teeth. Poor circulation and cold extremities, evidenced by chilblains, suggest a need for Calc Phos. It may assist with poor digestion, for example, if there is heartburn, indigestion or poor appetite.

Calc Phos, together with Mag Phos, may help relieve backache and headache during pregnancy. Use it if you have a history of dental problems or insufficient calcium intake.

Calc Sulph   (Calcium Sulphate)

Keywords: **Cleanser, purifier**
Preferences: **Likes fresh air**
              Hates damp weather

Calc Sulph aids effective cleansing of toxins by the body. It does this throughout the body but especially in the liver, which is the major organ responsible for filtering and disposing of toxic materials in the system. Therefore, use it whenever there is some cleansing to be done. This may be a sinus infection, a nasal discharge, acne or boils. Any discharge that is yellow suggests a need for Calc Sulph.

Ferr Phos   (Iron Phosphate)

Keywords: **Infection, anaemia**
Preferences: **Likes cold on the inflamed part and**
              warmth elsewhere
              Dislikes too much movement
              Often worse at night

Iron is needed for the production of haemoglobin, an important constituent of our blood responsible for carrying oxygen around our bodies. Lack of iron leads to anaemia, tiredness, listlessness and pallor.

It is also needed for the production of antibodies, and, therefore, is involved in our immune response to infection. Due to this involvement of iron in antibody production, Ferr Phos is useful whenever there is any infection or inflammation. It seems to be most effective in the very early stages.

Iron is not stored in our bodies for long, so women are especially prone to iron deficiency due to their regular blood loss during menstruation. Men generally need less iron than women. Assimilation of iron is often a problem, and in these cases Ferr Phos is invaluable as it helps you to absorb your iron and assimilate it correctly. Consider using it if your iron supplement causes side effects. The side effects suggest that your body is not assimilating the iron. (Note that iron absorption also needs vitamin C.)

Ferr Phos is a particularly useful tissue salt during pregnancy as it can be used in the early stages of a cold or flu to prevent a more serious condition developing. It also helps absorption of iron from your food and your supplement.

Kali Mur   (Potassium Chloride)

Keywords: **Thick, white discharges**
Preferences: **Hates rich, fatty food**

A need for Kali Mur is characterised by thick, white discharges. This may describe phlegm in the respiratory system, for example, sinus or nasal discharges, or mucus in the throat. Glandular swellings associated with colds and sore throats suggest Kali Mur. Kali Mur is often given with Ferr Phos in the early stages of an infection. The Kali Mur helps the early white discharge, and the Ferr Phos helps with fighting the infection. If the discharge becomes yellow, indicating deeper infection, use Calc Sulph or Kali Sulph in place of the Kali Mur.

Kali Phos   (Potassium Phosphate)

Keywords: **Nerve nutrient**
Preferences: **Needs rest, warmth**
              Hates exertion, cold

Potassium regulates nerve transmission and helps the muscles to respond to nerve impulses. When combined in Kali Phos, it has a strong effect on the nervous system. It is especially useful in any condition where there is weakness, nervousness, irritability or lethargy. In contrast to the anaemia and lethargy of Ferr Phos, the exhaustion of Kali Phos is related to depletion by living on one's nerves. This may be demonstrated by sleeplessness, headaches after overwork, weakness in the arms and legs after overexertion, or any general feeling of nervousness. Use during or after pregnancy any time you feel overwhelmed, overworked or overtired. Straight after the birth Kali Phos encourages a feeling of calm and will help you relax.

Kali Sulph (Potassium Sulphate)

Keywords: Yellow discharges, skin complaints
Preferences: Hates overheated rooms

Kali Sulph affects the skin and all mucous membranes such as the lining tissue of the throat. It has the mucousy properties of Kali Mur, but the mucus has become more chronic and yellow in colour and may be offensive. Long lasting sinus conditions, chronic catarrh of the nose, throat or middle ear may all suggest Kali Sulph. If the skin is affected, there may be scaling and possibly also a discharge.

Mag Phos (Magnesium Phosphate)

Keywords: Spasms, cramps
Preferences: Likes to be warm
Likes pressure on the affected area
Hates the cold

Magnesium is important for your nervous system, the heart, your bones and muscles. Mag Phos is useful for any sort of spasm or tension due to nervous system or muscular overactivity. For example, spasms or cramps associated with premenstrual syndrome or ovulation, cramps in the legs or a nervous stomach involving spasms may respond to Mag Phos. It is especially useful during the third trimester of pregnancy when cramps may be common because of the increased need for magnesium. Taken together with Calc Phos it helps to relieve many cases of backache or headache.

Prevention of osteoporosis depends on magnesium as well as on calcium. Therefore, ensure that you have adequate amounts of magnesium in the diet and its adequate assimilation by using Mag Phos.

Nat Mur   (Sodium Chloride)

Keywords: **Fluid disturbances**
Preferences: **Likes open air, hates heat**

Sodium chloride, or common table salt, has been linked to oedema or fluid retention. Therefore, any condition involving a fluid imbalance such as fluid retention or dryness of any membranes may respond to Nat Mur's balancing effect on the absorption of sodium chloride. It can be used even if salt is being restricted in the diet, as it does not contribute to a salt load; rather, it helps the body to use salt correctly to maintain the appropriate moisture balance throughout the body.

Nat Phos   (Sodium Phosphate)

Keywords: **Acid balance**
Preferences: **Hates weather changes**
                    Hates fatty foods

This is a great remedy for any state of acidity. This may be from an acid stomach, heartburn, sour vomiting, or arthritic conditions as a result of acid build-up in the body. Nat Phos is useful if you experience reflux or a feeling that food keeps coming back up, especially if there is a burning feeling. General vague feelings of nausea will often respond to Nat Phos.

Nat Sulph (Sodium Sulphate)

Keywords: **Water imbalance**
Preferences: **Hates dampness**
              Likes dry weather

Nat Sulph is another remedy which helps with digestion by its effect on the liver and production of bile. In supporting liver function the remedy can be used for nausea, a bitter taste in the mouth, biliousness or flatulence. Oedema may also be present anywhere in the body.

Silica

Keywords: **Toxin eliminator**
Preferences: **Likes to be warm**
              Hates the cold

Silica strengthens all the structures of the body – it supports weak ligaments, tendons and bones. It gives strong nail growth, and a lack of Silica will manifest as brittle or ingrown nails. Hair and skin also need Silica for strength and integrity.

Silica is useful wherever the strength of tissue is compromised in expelling foreign material, such as fragments of glass or rose thorns that have become embedded. Used in acne or other skin complaints, where the problem lies just below the surface, Silica will bring the problem quickly to resolution. Any skin problem that is slow to heal, such as boils and acne, may benefit from the use of Silica along with other remedies.

Calc Fluor and Silica often work together to maintain the strength and integrity of tissue: Calc Fluor is used to strengthen tissue and Silica to nourish and maintain integrity of the area. Use both to prevent cracked nipples.

Using the Tissue Salts

Choose the tissue salt which best matches the problem. You can use two or three together, but if you feel that you need more or or if you are finding it hard to limit your choices, it may be best to seek professional help. Combinations of various tissue salts are available for specific conditions and may be useful if many tissue salts seem to be indicated.

To use the tissue salts, you need to distinguish between acute and chronic conditions. Acute conditions generally come on suddenly and tend to be quite strong in their presentation. For example, a flu which hits suddenly would be classed as an acute condition. Acute conditions usually require use of the tissue salts frequently. So, if you have the flu, you would need to take the tissue salt or salts every half-hour for the first few hours. Then reduce the dose gradually until you are taking one tablet four times a day towards the end of the flu. You will probably need to take a flu remedy only for about one week.

Chronic conditions tend to come on more slowly and be longer lasting. For example, skin complaints are generally chronic, as they evolve slowly and last for long periods of time. Chronic conditions will often benefit from frequent early dosing, followed by regular but less frequent use. In acne the combination of Kali Mur, Kali Sulph, Calc Sulph and Silica should be taken every hour for the first two days, followed by four times a day as long as it is necessary. This may be quite a long time in some cases. Allow two to three months for best results.

To take the tissue salts, dissolve under the tongue or chew one or two at a time. They may be dissolved in warm water if preferred.

If you notice no improvement in a few hours for acute problems or in a few days or weeks in chronic cases, change the remedy or seek professional advice.

Chapter 11

MODALITIES AND THERAPIES

This chapter gives a brief overview of the various modalities used in this book. While the emphasis here is on their value during pregnancy, these modalities can be used to help with a wide variety of complaints at any time during your life. You can purchase many of the remedies recommended in this book and use them yourself, but it is always beneficial if you understand their mode of action. If you need a practitioner, this section will give you an idea of the various practitioners, what they do and how they practise. You will then be able to choose the best modality or combination of modalities for your circumstances.

ACUPUNCTURE

This technique is becoming more widely known and respected. Acupuncturists use specific points on the body, the acupuncture points, to stimulate healing. Don't be put off by the thought of the needles because many practitioners now use a laser instead. This is painless, but still effective.

The Therapeutic Goods Administration has the role of approving drugs for use by Australians. This body has a Traditional Medicine Evaluation Committee responsible for evaluating the effectiveness of herbs and other traditional forms of medicine such as acupuncture. Chinese medicine is offered at some universities and Traditional Chinese Medicine (TCM) has recently been registered in Victoria to standardise course content and educational requirements, to report adverse events and to develop consistent codes of professional conduct. Other Australian States are expected to follow the Victorian model for TCM.

Acupuncture is very successful in treating a range of conditions, including morning sickness, backache and headaches, and overdue and slow labour, to name a few. Complaints that are long-standing and not able to be treated by western medicine often respond to acupuncture.

Usually you need to have a few sessions, especially if the complaint is long-standing. However, some complaints respond very quickly and you may need only one or two treatments.

BACH FLOWER REMEDIES AND OTHER FLOWER ESSENCES

Flower remedies are prescribed for emotional rather than physical states. They can have a deep impact on feelings of wellbeing and bring a feeling of peace, calm and balance to distressed minds. The best-known, the Bach flower remedies, are discussed extensively in chapter 9.

They are safe and non-toxic to use. They are especially effective for babies and very young children. A drop of the remedy for shock immediately after birth will help the newborn to dispel any negative experience from the birth.

BOWEN THERAPY

Developed by an Australian chiropractor, Bowen therapy is a very gentle technique that moves soft tissue to stimulate healing in the damaged area. Safe and effective for all age groups, including the newborn and the very old, the technique has been successful in treating conditions such as knee and back pain, migraines, carpal tunnel syndrome and neck pain. It is also very balancing and calming. Many people find that they sleep better after a Bowen treatment, they deal more effectively with stress and generally just feel better.

Most problems will resolve with just a few treatments, but regular Bowen treatments can keep you feeling well and in control of your life. This is especially true if you have a stressful job or many stressful events in your life.

HERBALISM

Herbalists and naturopaths use plants in various forms. These may be the flower, the bark of a tree or the root of the plant. Herbs have a long tradition of use, and herbs from many countries are now becoming more widely available. Chinese, Indian and North American herbs are all used regularly in Australia.

Some ingredients have been extracted from herbs and used as the basis of some of our modern drugs. Notably, digitalis, a drug used for serious heart conditions, is extracted from the herb foxglove. Herbalists believe that the whole plant is better therapeutically than an extract, as the plant contains balancing ingredients which reduce any toxic effects. For example, celery is a diuretic, that is, it encourages urination and increases the output of urine. Celery is also high in potassium, which often needs to be replaced in people on pharmaceutical diuretics. Therefore, the natural diuretic action of celery is balanced in the plant by its high potassium content. Generally herbs are more normalising than pharmaceutical drugs. For example, they will balance hormones or blood pressure and will not raise them or lower them to extreme values.

Many herbs are quite safe to use during pregnancy and are gentle and effective. Many of the herbs recommended in this book are easily available from health food stores. If you wish to use these herbs, use them only for the recommended purpose and follow the dosage given on the container. This will ensure that you are using a safe dose of the herb. Other herbs are available only from qualified herbalists and naturopaths. See my Author's Note for a discussion of the safety of herbs during pregnancy and lactation.

A herbalist or naturopath will choose a combination of a few herbs to suit your circumstances. Usually you need to take them regularly for a period of time to obtain the best results. Some problems resolve quickly, but others will need ongoing treatment.

HOMOEOPATHY

Homoeopathic remedies are prepared using minute doses of the substance required. Therefore, they are safe and non-toxic and, if used correctly, there are no side effects.

Homoeopathic preparations are available from health food stores to cover a range of everyday conditions. These include sleeplessness, sinus problems, hay fever and flu. There are also some combinations especially prepared for infants and very young children. Remedies for colic, teething and stomach disturbances are safe and effective ways of dealing with these conditions. Arnica, used for bruising and after injury, is available as drops to take by mouth or as a cream to rub in. It is recommended after birth for both mother and baby. It is a great remedy to have if you have accident-prone children.

Always follow the recommended dosage for your homoeopathic remedy unless directed otherwise by a trained homoeopath or naturopath. Once the symptoms have abated you generally do not need to continue using the remedy unless otherwise directed.

There are many homoeopathic remedies, so the field is quite complex. Homoeopaths will usually question you about your lifestyle and your health history to determine the best remedy for you. They will then match your symptoms with the correct homoeopathic remedy. As there are very many remedies to choose from, homoeopaths need to be very specific to select the correct one. Homoeopathy is not useful just when you are ill, it can be used to help build resistance. Homoeopathic vaccination kits have been developed as a suggested alternative to pharmaceutical vaccination.

MASSAGE THERAPY

Massage no longer has the bad reputation it once did. Massage is a valuable therapeutic tool. It can be used to relax, to soothe sore and aching muscles, or to treat sports injuries. The massage recommended in this book is mostly relaxation, with some remedial applications. Other forms of massage include Shiatsu, Oriental, Swedish, deep tissue and sports massage.

When choosing a massage therapist, make sure that he or she belongs to a recognised association. If you are a little wary or nervous, make a half-hour appointment to start with. Your next visit can be longer if you choose. Some naturopaths also offer massage and this can be very useful if you also need to discuss nutritional requirements. A naturopath might also recommend herbs or other supplements which can help with various aches and pains.

NATUROPATHY

Naturopaths use a variety of methods to help you. They have studied herbs, Bach flowers, tissue salts, diet, homoeopathy, vitamins and minerals. Some practise massage and/or Bowen therapy as well. They will discuss your diet and lifestyle, as well as any health problems you are experiencing.

A naturopath might make recommendations involving changes to your lifestyle such as dietary changes. These are best regarded as long-term goals, with the ultimate aim of making some permanent changes. Any supplements you are given may be recommended on an ongoing basis, depending on the nature of the problem. During pregnancy, however, as your body is changing so quickly, you may need some of these only for short periods of time.

OSTEOPATHY

A manual therapy, osteopathy treats the joints and muscles to restore body movement and to remove restrictions to healing. Osteopaths believe that many health problems, not just muscular or skeletal problems, can be attributed to an area of disordered mechanical structure. Areas of tension may be treated with deep pressure, stretching and manipulation.

For the mother during her pregnancy, the changing weight distribution and the effect of relaxing ligaments may lead to backache. Pre-existing complaints, such as some forms of arthritis, may flare up during pregnancy. These problems often respond easily to osteopathic. treatment. Treatment during pregnancy is gentle and light. Osteopathic treatment is not necessarily forceful manipulation of bones and joints. Osteopaths use gentle soft tissue techniques, stretching and mobilisation to restore balance to the body. There are also techniques to encourage labour if the pregnancy has gone past term.

Cranial osteopathy has been developed to work gently with the bones of the skull to maintain normal position and movement. The bones of the skull or cranium should be free to move very slightly. Restriction to this movement may result from injury as a result of pressure during a long or difficult birth. The baby's head is often misshapen due to the tremendous forces experienced during birth. Injury may also result from internal trauma during the pregnancy, from a fall or a car accident. Symptoms which might suggest restriction to the normal small movement of the skull bones include colic, unexplained crying, sleep difficulties, difficulties in feeding and recurrent ear infections. Because the movement of the cranial bones is very slight, cranial techniques are gentle and very relaxing. Cranial osteopathy is suitable for very young babies, who generally respond very well to the technique.

REIKI

Reiki is a system of energy healing that is becoming more widely known and respected. It is a very simple yet effective way of generating balance, calm and support. Therapists of any discipline can become Reiki channels, and you might find massage therapists, midwives and naturopaths using Reiki. Reiki may help to remove emotional blocks to good health and wellbeing.

During pregnancy, Reiki can be used to balance emotions when you feel out-of-sorts, overwhelmed or confused by the changes happening to you. Fear of the birth itself is not unusual, especially in first-time mothers. Reiki sessions will help to bring out these fears and give you confidence in your ability to deal with labour and birth. Similarly, any fear of the responsibilities involved in parenthood can be addressed during a Reiki session. A Reiki session usually lasts about an hour and is very relaxing and comforting. Generally you will lie down during the session, close your eyes and the practitioner will place his or her hands in various positions to transfer the Reiki energy to your body.

Reiki is very effective for babies. After a Reiki session a baby will sleep well and will be calmer and happier.

SCHUESSLER TISSUE SALTS

Tissue salts are minerals which form the basis of our bodies. The Schuessler tissue salts are prepared using very small amounts of the mineral to form a dilute powder dispersed through a tablet medium. This small concentration of the mineral enables the body to better assimilate the particular mineral being used. The tissue salts help the body to compensate for deficiencies in absorption or digestion and to restore balance where appropriate.

The low concentrations used make the tissue salts very safe to use. There are no toxic side effects.

In an acute condition, such as a cold or flu, the tissue salts can be taken or chewed regularly every twenty to thirty minutes if necessary. Avoid strong tastes or odours around the time you use the tissue salts. If you have just brushed your teeth or chewed some gum, wait about fifteen minutes before using the tissue salts. They are best chewed rather than swallowed.

For long-standing conditions , tissue salts are generally recommended four times each day.

Tissue salts are available from health food stores. For a full description of each of the tissue salts see chapter 10. There are also some combinations available for a variety of problems, such as hay fever, after injury, for sinus or skin problems. Tissue salts can be very effective and are safe and easy to use. If you need to have tissue salts prescribed for you, you would need to see a naturopath or a homoeopath.

AVAILABILITY OF SUGGESTED REMEDIES

Many of the remedies suggested in this book are readily available from health food stores. Take this book with you to ensure that you get exactly the right remedy. Check the dosage before you leave the store to ensure that you know exactly how much to take or how to use the remedy. Many health food stores now have a naturopath in attendance if you need any extra help or advice.

Some of the recommended remedies need to be obtained from a qualified naturopath, herbalist or homoeopath, who will give you valuable advice and ensure that your good health plan is complete and balanced.

AVAILABILITY OF THERAPISTS

For a therapist near you, it is best to check in your local telephone directory. Make sure that the therapist is a member of a recognised association. This ensures that he or she has recognised training and qualifications. Therapists are listed either under their association's heading in the phone book, or they will nominate their association membership and credentials in their personal listing.

Acupuncture

Acupuncture Association of Victoria Ltd
Enquiries   (03) 9557 6100

Australian Acupuncture Association Ltd
National Administration   1800 025 334

Aromatherapy

Many massage therapists also practise aromatherapy. Some
naturopaths have experience with essential oils.

International Federation of Aromatherapists Inc (Aust)
P.O. Box 467
Hurstbridge   VIC   3099   1902 240 125

Bowen Therapy

Bowen Therapists Association of Victoria   (03) 9809 0688
Other states will soon have telephone listings.
Many naturopaths and massage therapists also practise Bowen
therapy. Sometimes this may be stipulated in their telephone
listing, but you may need to ring some local therapists to find
one that has the combination of modalities you need, including
Bowen therapy.

Herbalism

National Herbalists Association of Australia
305/3 Small Street
Broadway   NSW   2007   (02) 9211 6437

Victorian Herbalists Association
P.O. Box 205
Clifton Hill   VIC   3068   014 868 461

Homoeopathy

Australian Homoeopathic Association
40 Rangeview Road
St Andrews   VIC   3761   (03) 9710 1606

Homoeopathic Education and Research Association
151 Union Street
Windsor   VIC   3181   (03) 9521 2779

Victorian Register of Certified Homoeopathic Practitioners
3 Willow Street
Preston   VIC   3072   (03) 9484 6048

Massage Therapy

Association of Massage Therapists Australia (Inc)
250 High Street
Prahran   VIC   3181   (03) 9510 3930

Naturopathy

Australian Natural Therapists Association Ltd
National Administration Office
P.O. Box 856
Caloundra   QLD   4551   1800 817 577

Australian Traditional Medicine Society
Head Office
Unit 12/27 Bank Street
Meadowbank   NSW   2114   (02) 9809 6800

Osteopathy

Australian Osteopathic Association
Federal Office
P.O. Box 699
Turramurra   NSW   2074   (02) 9449 4799

Victorian State Office
109 Canterbury Road
Bayswater   VIC   3153   (03) 9720 7970

Reiki

Reiki therapists do not have a special listing in the telephone directory. Many therapists who specialise in other areas may also practise Reiki. You may find masseurs, naturopaths and nurses with Reiki training. There are also a few medical practitioners who are Reiki practitioners as well. This may or may not be advertised, but if you wish to experience Reiki, ask your therapist if he or she offers it.

GLOSSARY

Acidophilus (also known as lactobacillus acidophilus) is the most plentiful of the beneficial bacteria living in the digestive system. It contributes to good digestion and prevents overgrowth of harmful bacteria.

Amniotic fluid is the fluid surrounding and protecting the developing foetus. Some is swallowed by the foetus. 'Breaking the waters' refers to the natural or artificial rupturing of the membrane which encloses the baby and the amniotic fluid. This allows the escape of the amniotic fluid and usually hastens labour.

Antioxidants protect against the damaging effects of free radicals from environmental pollutants, pesticides, cigarette smoke etc. Antioxidants include the vitamins A, C and E as well as several herbs such as green tea and grape seed extract.

Arachidonic acid is a fatty acid produced by our bodies and found in animal products.

Areola (plural areolae) is the pink or brown tissue surrounding the nipple.

Aromatherapy uses essential oils prepared from plants. The healing properties of the plant are concentrated in the essential oil. The oils contain hundreds of constituents, which combine to give essential oils an array of therapeutic properties.

Bifidobacterium infantis is the predominant probiotic in the digestive tract of infants and young children.

Bifidus (also known as bifidobacteria) is the beneficial bacteria living in the digestive system and contributing to good digestion and the inhibition of harmful bacteria.

Braxton Hicks contractions occur in late pregnancy, but may be misinterpreted as true labour. They may be very powerful, and may partly dilate the cervix.

Caesarean section involves delivery of the baby through the abdominal wall. It may be performed if the mother or baby is at risk.

Candida albicans is a yeast-like fungus that lives in the digestive system. It may proliferate, leading to symptoms of thrush, allergy and digestive disturbances. This may happen as a result of poor diet, antibiotic use, poor immune response or stress.

Carbohydrates are the main energy source in our food supply, being converted to glucose by the digestive process. Produced by plants, carbohydrate foods include grains, fruits and vegetables, and legumes or pulses.

Cervix is the lower part of the uterus, forming a narrow passage connecting with the vagina. It must dilate about 10 cm during labour to allow passage of the baby.

Cholesterol is a vital component of the membranes of our cells. It is produced from fats by all animals. While it is a necessary ingredient of our bodies, too much can be harmful, contributing to heart and artery disease.

Colostrum is the first secretion of the breasts, before the milk starts. It is clear and watery and contains protective antibodies.

Conception occurs when the sperm from the male and the

ovum (egg) from the female unite, forming the early beginnings of an embryo.

Cravings for strange foods or combinations of foods are common in pregnancy. They may be related to mineral or other nutrient deficiencies.

Dilation of the cervix occurs during the first stage of labour to allow room for the passage of the baby through the birth canal.

Diuretics increase the output of urine.

Embryo. The developing baby is called an embryo from the beginning of week four until the end of week eight.

Epidural anaesthesia is anaesthetic injected into the spinal cord to numb sensation in the lower part of the body.

Episiotomy is the surgical enlargement of the vaginal opening. Performed under a local anaesthetic, it requires later repair with stitches.

Essential fatty acids. Fatty acids are the main components of the cell walls and the fats in our bodies. The essential fatty acids must be obtained from the diet. These are linoleic acid, linolenic acid and arachidonic acid. Sources of essential fatty acids include nuts and seeds, linseeds and their oil, evening primrose oil and fish oil.

Essential oils are the concentrated extracts from plants. They are liquids but are not oily at all. Some oils are very expensive due to the low yield from the plant material. They need to be diluted before use.

Fat is a concentrated energy source. Some fat is essential in the diet, but too much contributes to obesity and heart disease.

Fats may be monounsaturated, polyunsaturated or saturated. Generally, fresh polyunsaturated and monounsaturated fats are beneficial. Saturated fats are the fats that have been implicated in causing disease.

Fibre may be soluble or insoluble. Both types are essential for proper functioning of the bowel and good digestion.

Foetus refers to the developing baby after the beginning of the ninth week.

Folic acid is one of the B group of vitamins. Its name is derived from foliage, meaning leaf. It has a number of functions as do all vitamins. Essential for the developing embryo, it is often supplemented before pregnancy and during the first trimester.

Forceps are designed to grasp and fit snugly around the baby's head to enable the extraction of the foetus, if the mother is unable to push the baby out herself.

Free radicals are byproducts of metabolism and are found in environmental pollutants, cigarette smoke, etc. They are highly unstable, able to damage cells and are believed to be implicated in the pathogenesis of many diseases, including some cancers.

Haemorrhoids (piles) are enlarged areas in the veins around the anus. In pregnancy, they are the result of constipation and relaxation of the blood vessel walls due to hormonal changes. They often bleed and may be painless or quite painful.

Lanugo is the fine hair that covers the foetus. Formed from the sixteenth week, it has usually disappeared by the expected date of delivery.

Linoleic acid, a polyunsaturated fatty acid, is one of the essential fatty acids required for life. It is found in many nuts and seeds and in evening primrose oil.

Linolenic acid, also known as alpha-linolenic acid, is an essential fatty acid. It is found in green plants, linseed oil, nuts and seeds.

Mastitis, or breast inflammation, may develop during breast-feeding as a result of bacteria introduced through cracked nipples.

Meconium is the name given to the baby's first bowel contents. It is dark green or black, and contains bile pigments and other metabolic debris. Meconium in the amniotic fluid suggests foetal distress.

Minerals make up the earth. Many are essential for our growth and development. These include calcium, magnesium, iron and zinc. Due to our farming practices, many minerals have been removed from our food supply and not replaced. This has led to deficiencies. Processing may further reduce the mineral content of foods.

Monounsaturated fat is necessary for proper development of the cell membrane and protects against heart disease and high cholesterol levels.

Ovulation involves the release of a mature egg (ovum) which then travels down the fallopian tube. The mature ovum is able to be fertilised in the tube, resulting in conception.

Perineum is the area between the anus and the vaginal opening. This is cut when an episiotomy is performed.

Placenta attaches the foetus to the wall of the uterus. It is the source of nourishment for the developing foetus. The placenta also removes waste products and carries oxygen to the foetus.

Polyunsaturated fat is essential as it is a source of the essential fatty acids. Polyunsaturated fats are easily converted to toxic products by heating and processing. Only fresh and unprocessed foods contain the essential fatty acids. Polyunsaturated fats are able to return cholesterol and saturated fats to the liver for processing and are therefore protective against heart disease and obesity.

Pre-eclampsia (toxaemia) affects some mothers in late pregnancy. High blood pressure, oedema and the presence of protein in the urine suggest pre-eclampsia. It may develop into eclampsia, a serious condition for mother and baby.

Probiotics are the beneficial bacteria which colonise the digestive system. They include lactobacillus acidophilus and bifidobacteria.

Protein is composed of amino acids. Eight amino acids are essential for adults, and ten for children. These must be obtained from the diet. The other 14 amino acids can be made by the body if we have adequate amounts of the essential ones. Protein is essential for growth and repair of body tissue. Protein can be obtained from a variety of plant and animal sources.

Saturated fat is found in animal products such as meat and dairy foods. Many processed and fast foods contain high levels of saturated fats. Saturated fats are not essential to health and have been implicated in a variety of diseases such as obesity and heart disease.

Stretch marks occur when the skin does not have sufficient elasticity to grow quickly during periods of rapid growth such as pregnancy. Initially they may be quite dark, but will fade over the years.

Thrush is caused by candida albicans, a yeast-like fungus that lives in the digestive system. It may affect the mouth or vagina. Symptoms include white patches on the cheeks or tongue if the mouth is affected. If the vagina is affected there may be itching, discharge or damage to the external skin.

Toxaemia (see pre-eclampsia)

Triglycerides are the fats our bodies use as stored energy. As well as storing energy and essential fatty acids for use by the body, they are necessary for insulating and protecting our bodies.

Umbilical cord connects the baby to the mother's uterus. It transports nutrient-rich blood to the developing baby and returns metabolic byproducts to be disposed by the mother's system.

Uterus (womb) is the baby's home for the first nine months of life. It expands during pregnancy, to allow implantation and development of the placenta. At the end of the pregnancy, the uterine muscles contract to expel the foetus and placenta.

Vernix is an oily layer covering the foetus to protect the skin.

Vitamins are essential for our growth and development. They include the fat-soluble vitamins A, D, E and K, as well as the water-soluble vitamins B and C. The water-soluble vitamins must be obtained every day. Highly processed foods contain few vitamins and cooking destroys many vitamins.

QUICK REFERENCE GUIDE

PROBLEM	TISSUE SALT	HERBS	VITAMINS & MINERALS	BACH FLOWERS	AROMA-THERAPY	OTHER
Backache	Calc Phos Mag Phos					Massage Bowen therapy Osteopathy
Braxton Hicks contractions		Squaw vine False unicorn root Black haw Cramp back				Frequent rest
Breast engorgement	Kali Mur	Dandelion root			Geranium oil Rose oil Lavender oil	
Carpel tunnel syndrome			Vitamin B6			Bowen therapy
Colds and flu	Ferr Phos, Kali Mur Kali or Calc Sulph	Echinacea Garlic	Vitamin C		Eucalyptus oil Tea tree oil	Homoeopathic preparations Plenty of rest Plenty of fluids

PROBLEM	TISSUE SALT	HERBS	VITAMINS & MINERALS	BACH FLOWERS	AROMA-THERAPY	OTHER
Colic		Chamomile Peppermint Fennel	Bifidobacterium Infantis		Chamomile oil Peppermint oil Fennel oil	Check feeding technique Tummy massage Osteopathic treatment Homoeopathic preparations
Constipation	Ferr Phos if caused by iron supplement					Fibre Exercise Plenty of fluids
Cracked nipples	Ferr Phos Calc Fluor Silica	Calendula cream Echinacea Garlic Vitamin C				Honey Air nipples
Cradle cap		Hamamelis Wild Pansy cream	(for mother) Essential fatty acids Linseed oil Evening primrose & fish oils		Chamomile oil	

PROBLEM	TISSUE SALT	HERBS	VITAMINS & MINERALS	BACH FLOWERS	AROMA-THERAPY	OTHER
Cramps	Mag Phos Calc Phos		Magnesium			Massage Exercise
Cravings			all minerals			
Dental problems	Calc Phos Mag Phos		Calcium Magnesium Vitamin C			Regular flossing Regular dental checks
Dry skin		Calendula cream	(for mother) Essential fatty acids Linseed oil Evening primrose & fish oils		Chamomile oil	
Episiotomy			Zinc Vitamin A Vitamin E		Lavender oil	Homoeopathic Arnica
Faintness			Vitamin E			

PROBLEM	TISSUE SALT	HERBS	VITAMINS & MINERALS	BACH FLOWERS	AROMA-THERAPY	OTHER
Fatigue			B vitamins Iron Fresh foods			Frequent rest
Fluid retention		Celery Dandelion leaf	Vitamin B6			Exercise Avoid salty foods
Groin pain						Bowen therapy
Haemorrhoids		Hamamelis ointment				Exercise Fibre Plenty of fluids
Headaches	Calc Phos Mag Phos					Bowen therapy Osteopathy Massage Check for allergies

PROBLEM	TISSUE SALT	HERBS	VITAMINS & MINERALS	BACH FLOWERS	AROMA-THERAPY	OTHER
Indigestion		Chamomile Peppermint				Eat small frequent meals Homoeopathic Nux vomica
Insufficient milk		Blessed thistle Agnus castus Raspberry leaves	Complete nutrition	Rescue Remedy Appropriate Bach flowers	Clary sage oil Geranium oil	Avoid tea, coffee Obtain plenty rest
Labour		Blue cohosh Black cohosh Cramp back Raspberry leaves Motherwort		Rescue Remedy	Clary sage oil Petitgrain oil Neroli oil Lavender oil Rose oil Geranium oil Sandalwood oil Tangerine oil Ylang ylang	Massage Compresses Music Bath Homoeopathic Caulophyllum

PROBLEM	TISSUE SALT	HERBS	VITAMINS & MINERALS	BACH FLOWERS	AROMA-THERAPY	OTHER
Labour preparation		Raspberry leaves Squaw vine False unicorn root Black haw Cramp bark	Complete nutrition	Rescue Remedy Aspen Clematis Gentian Hornbeam Mimulus Wild Oat Walnut	Chamomile oil Eucalyptus oil Geranium oil Lavender oil Neroli oil Rose oil	Massage Bowen therapy Music Reiki
Mastitis	Ferr Phos Kali Mur Silica	Dandelion root tea Garlic Echinacea	Vitamin C	Rescue Remedy		Aloe vera gel topically
Morning sickness	Kali Mur Nat Phos	Chamomile Peppermint Ginger	Vitamin B6			Eat small frequent meals Homoeopathic Nux vomica

PROBLEM	TISSUE SALT	HERBS	VITAMINS & MINERALS	BACH FLOWERS	AROMA-THERAPY	OTHER
Nappy rash		Pawpaw cream Chamomile	Zinc cream Essential fatty acids (for mother) Linseed oil Evening primrose & fish oils (for mother) Bifidobacterium infantis		Chamomile oil	
Postnatal depression		St John's wort Agnus castus	Complete nutrition	Rescue Remedy Appropriate Bach flowers	Neroli oil Petitgrain oil	Exercise Support Plenty of rest
Skin problems			(for mother) Essential fatty acids Linseed oil Evening primrose & fish oils			
Sleepless baby		Chamomile		Rescue Remedy Appropriate Bach flowers	Lavender oil	Ensure baby is warm, fed, does not have colic Play music Osteopathy

PROBLEM	TISSUE SALT	HERBS	VITAMINS & MINERALS	BACH FLOWERS	AROMA-THERAPY	OTHER
Sleep disturbances	Kali Phos	Chamomile Hops Valerian Passionflower			Lavender oil	Massage Avoid coffee
Stretch marks			Zinc Vitamin E cream & supplement		Neroli oil Lavender oil Tangerine oil	Massage with jojoba oil
Thrush			Acidophilus & bifidus (mother) Bifidobacterium infantis (baby)			Avoid sweet foods Homoeopathic preparations
Umbilical cord		Echinacea (dilute)			Oil of cloves (dilute)	
Varicose veins			Hamamelis			Elevate legs whenever possible Gentle exercise

REFERENCES

Nutrition

Aharoni A, Tesler B, Paltieli Y, Tal J, Dori Z and Sharf M, 'Hair chromium content of women with gestational diabetes compared with nondiabetic pregnant women', *American Journal of Clinical Nutrition*, 1992, 55:104-107.

Australian Council for Responsible Nutrition, *Vitamins and Minerals: Functions and Safety*, July 1998.

Barrett B M, Sowell A, Gunter E and Wang M, 'Potential role of ascorbic acid and beta-carotene in the prevention of preterm rupture of foetal membranes', *International Journal for Vitamin and Nutrition Research*, 1994, 64(3):192-7.

Barrington J W, Lindsay P, James D, Smith S and Roberts A, 'Selenium deficiency and miscarriage: a possible link', *British Journal of Obstetrics and Gynecology*, 1996, 103:130-132.

Bekaroglu M, Aslan Y, Gedik Y, Deger O, Mocan H, Erduran and Karahan C, 'Relationships between serum free fatty acids and zinc, and attention deficit hyperactivity disorder: a research note', *Journal of Child Psychology and Psychiatry and Allied Disciplines*, 1996, 37:225-227.

Berger S M, *How To Be Your Own Nutritionist*, Bantam Books, Australia, 1987.

Bland J, *Medical Applications of Clinical Nutrition*, Keats Publishing, Connecticut, 1993.

Blaurock-Busch E, with Griffin V, *Minerals and Trace Element Analysis*, TMI, Boulder, Colorado, 1996.

Botto L D, Koury M J, Mulinare J and Erickson J D, 'Periconceptual multivitamin use and the occurrence of conotruncal heart defects: results from a population based, case-control study', *Pediatrics*, 1996-98, 911-917.

Bung P, Prinz-Langenohl R, Thorand B and Pietrzik K, 'Micronutrients during pregnancy: the nutritive situation in

Germany', *Asia-Pacific Journal of Obstetrics and Gynecology*, 1996, 103:130-132.

Dahle L O, 'The effect of oral magnesium substitution on pregnancy-induced leg cramps', *American Journal of Obstetrics and Gynecology*, 1995, 173(1):175-180.

Erasmus U, *Fats That Heal, Fats That Kill*, Alive Books, Canada, 1996.

Garg H K, 'Zinc taste test in pregnant women and its correlation with serum zinc level,' *Indian Journal of Physiology and Pharmacology*, 1993, 37(4): 318-322.

Gold S and Sherry L, 'Hyperactivity, learning disabilities, and alcohol,' *Journal of Learning Disabilities*, 1984, 17(1):3-6.

Guvenc H, Karatas F, Guvenc M, Kunc S, Aygun A D and Bektas S, 'Low levels of selenium in mothers and their newborns in pregnancies with a neural tube defect', *Pediatrics*, June, 1995, 95(6):879-882M.

Holman S R, *Essentials of Nutrition for the Health Professions*, J B Lappincott, Philadelphia, 1994.

Kock M U, *Laugh With Health*, Renaissance & New Age Creations, Australia, 1996.

Levine M, Conry-Cantilena C, Wang Y, Welsh R W, Washko P W, Dhariwal K R, Park J B, Lazarev A, Graumlich J F, King J and Cantilena L R, 'Vitamin C pharmacokinetics in healthy volunteers: evidence for a recommended dietary allowance', *Proceedings of the National Academy of Sciences of the United States of America*, 1996, 93(8):3704-9.

Mahomed K, James D, Golding J and McCabe R, 'Failure to taste zinc sulfate solution does not predict zinc deficiency in pregnancy', *European Journal of Obstetrics, Gynecology and Reproductive Biology*, 1993, 48(3): 169-175.

McCarron D A, 'Role of adequate dietary calcium intake in the prevention and management of salt-sensitive hypertension', *American Journal of Clinical Nutrition*, 1997, 65(suppl):712S-6S.

Mervyn L, *The Dictionary of Minerals*, Lothian Publishing, Northamptonshire, 1985.

Mindell E, *Food as Medicine*, Bookman Press, Melbourne, 1994.

Naish F and Roberts J, *The Natural Way to Better Babies*, Random House, Australia, 1996.

Nelson K B and Grether J K, 'Can Magnesium sulfate reduce the risk of cerebral palsy in very low birth weight infants?', *Pediatrics*, February 1995, 95(2):263-269.

Reece M S, McGregor J A, Allen K G D and Harris M A, 'Maternal and perinatal long-chain fatty acids: possible roles in preterm birth', *American Journal of Obstetrics and Gynecology*, 1997, 176(4):907-914.

Rondo P H C, Rodrigues L C and Tomkins A M, 'Coffee consumption and intrauterine growth retardation in Brazil', *European Journal of Clinical Nutrition*, 1996, 50(11): 705-9.

Tsukahara H, Deguchi Y, Hiraoka M, Hori C, Kimura K, Kawamitsu T, Konishi Y, Kusaka Y and Sudo M, 'Urinary selenium excretion in infancy: comparison between term and preterm infants', *Biology of the Neonate*, 1996, 70:35-40.

Werbach M R, *Nutritional Influences on Illness: A Sourcebook of Clinical Research*, Third Line Press, Tarzana, California, 1993.

Aromatherapy

England A, *Aromatherapy for Mother and Baby*, Random House, London 1993.

Schilcher H, *Phytotherapy in Paediatrics: Handbook for Physicians and Pharmacists*, Medpharm Scientific Publishers, 1997, Stuttgart.

Tisserand R, *The Art of Aromatherapy*, C W Daniel, Saffron Walden, England, 1998.

Tisserand R and Balacs T, *Essential Oil Safety: A Guide for Health Care Professionals*, Churchill Livingstone, Edinburgh, 1995.

Worwood V A, *The Fragrant Pharmacy*, Bantam Books, London 1995.

Bach Flower Remedies

Bach E, *Heal Thyself - An Explanation of the Real Cause & Cure of Disease*, C W Daniel, Saffron Walden, England, 1987.

Barnard J, *A Guide to the Bach Flower Remedies,* C W Daniel, Saffron Walden, England, 1987.

Chancellor P, *Handbook of the Bach Flower Remedies,* Keats Publishing, Connecticut, USA, 1971.

Herbs

Fischer-Rasmussen W, Kjaer S K, Dahl C and Asping U, 'Ginger treatment of hyperemesis gravidarum', *European Journal of Obstetrics, Gynecology and Reproductive Biology,* 1991, 38(1):19-24.

Hall D, *Dorothy Hall's Herbal Medicine,* Lothian Publishing, Australia, 1988.

Janssen P L T M K, Meyboom S, van Staveren W A, de Vegt F and Katan M B, 'Consumption of Ginger (Zingibar officinale Roscoe) does not affect ex vivo platelet thromboxane production in humans,' *European Journal of Clinical Nutrition,* 1996, 50:772-774.

Jorsal L, Lasskogen L and Weidner M S, *Review of Blood Thinning Effect of Ginger,* Institute of Drug Analysis, Copenhagen.

McIntyre A, *The Complete Woman's Herbal,* Gaia Books Ltd, London, 1995.

McIntyre A, *The Herbal for Mother and Child,* Element Books Ltd, Great Britain, 1992.

Murray M T, *The Healing Power of Herbs,* Prima Publishing, USA, 1995.

O'Connell J, *Traditional Herbal Compendium,* 1995.

Schilcher H, *Phytotherapy in Paediatrics: Handbook for Physicians and Pharmacists,* Medpharm Scientific Publishers,1997, Stuttgart.

Schuessler Tissue Salts

Boericke W, *Materia Medica with Repertory,* Jain, New Delhi , 1987.

Martin and Pleasance, *Handbook of the Biochemic Tissue Salts,* Melbourne, 1996.

Wells M, *The Tissue Salts,* Autonomy Books, Melbourne. 1995.

Other

Artal R, 'Exercise: an alternative therapy for gestational diabetes', *The Physician and Sportsmedicine*,1996, 24(3).

Bradford N and Williams J, *What They Don't Tell You about Being a Mother and Looking after Babies*, Harper Collins, London, 1997.

Golden I, *Vaccination*, Australia, 1998.

Kitzinger S, *The Complete Book of Pregnancy and Childbirth*, Dorling Kindersley, London, 1996.

Moore K L, *The Developing Human: Clinically Oriented Embryology*, W B Saunders, Harcourt Brace, USA, 1998.

O'Connor L J and Gourley R J, *Obstetric and Gynecological Care in Physical Therapy*, Slack, USA, 1990.

Olds S B, London M L and Ladewig P W, *Maternal Newborn Nursing: A Family-Centered Approach*, Fourth Edition, Addison-Wesley Nursing, Redwood City, California, 1992.

Stanway P and A, *Breast is Best*, Pan Books, London, 1983.

WHO Regional Publications, Western Pacific Series No. 2.

WHO Fact Sheet N 134, September 1996.

INDEX

g = Glossary

R = Quick Reference Guide